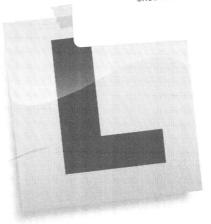

Immortality for Beginners

A crash course in health, happiness and eternal youth

By Peter Beard

Dea Chaion

I hope you enjoy this book.

Peter B~

Peter Beard
PUBLICATIONS

1 Wellgate • Old Glossop • Derbyshire SK13 7RS
author.beard@gmail.com

Editing and design by reverendpixel

ISBN 978-1480248274

2

About the author

Peter Beard lives for change. His first career was as a Chartered Accountant but, after discovering an affinity with computers, he became a computer programmer. For more than a decade he wrote specialist applications for international blue-chip companies until eventually he was introduced to a skincare clinic. This involvement led to a fascination for the way that modern technical advances were revolutionising the cosmetic skincare industry. He consequently founded SkinGenesis, his own skincare company, and for ten years he enthusiastically researched how to delay, and sometimes reverse, the manifestations of ageing.

Peter is also a certified NLP (neuro-linguistic programming) practitioner and now occupies his daylight hours mentoring and training; he still devotes any remaining time to increasing his understanding of the relationship between health, fitness and ageing. His involvement with SkinGenesis, together with his training experience and research, has convinced him that almost unlimited achievement is possible in life, irrespective of a person's age. To personally demonstrate this, he graded as a black belt in Mixed Martial Arts in 2011, a few months before his sixty-second birthday.

His philosophy is to wake each day in wonder at what life may bring, and that getting older is not a barrier but a means to making life better. There are a few simple rules that he follows to make this happen: Stay fit mentally, stay fit physically, stay positive and believe that everything is possible. It is also important to be going somewhere – providing it isn't down – unless of course you're skydiving!

For the collector of domestic statistics, he is currently married to the girl who first stole his heart when he was twenty-one, and together they have raised four children who continue to delight them.

Peter has appeared on television, and is a regular guest on BBC radio as a skin expert.

Contents

Preface

There is more to immortality than surviving a few more breaths and heartbeats while enduring an extra lap or two around the sun. It is about sowing a little thought and effort into your life, and in return reaping the rewards of extra health, happiness and fulfilment. It is about a holistic strategy for mind and body that will improve your health and fitness, as well as increase motivation and encourage a more positive outlook; it is how to live younger for longer. It is about acquiring what I call 'immortality'; it requires no previous experience, it is easy and inexpensive, and it makes life a lot of fun.

We all know immortals; persons with everlasting zest and an unquenchable enthusiasm for life; persons who have perpetual energy and who always anticipate the future with excitement. They are the ones who stay young while the world grows old around them.

Immortality requires your life to be both so fulfilling that you wake each morning wanting to live it a little longer, and also that you live your life in such a way that health, happiness and a few extra years are inevitable, rather than accidental. These requirements are mutually dependent, neither can happen without each other, and both sustain each other.

As I researched for this book, I found time and time again that as you put more effort into your life not only will you improve its quality, but you will also significantly increase your active life expectancy. I also found that performing a particular action will bring about general benefits beyond the intended specific and immediate benefits. For instance, exercising your body will improve your mood, health, cognitive abilities and life expectancy as well as the specific benefits of being fitter and physically more capable. To a large extent we are held back from seeking and achieving immortality by the barriers in our mind. These barriers are formed from our restricted expectation that, after reaching a certain age, we will begin an inevitable decline from which there is no return. Most of these expectations were handed down to us during our childhood by our parents and family and, unless we consciously take action to modify them, we are unlikely to ever reach our full potential.

My earliest recollection that people could be really old was when I first met my uncle Roger. Uncle Roger, or Roger the Dodger as my dad would call him, was still evading the military police, having spontaneously decided to take an unscheduled and unofficial vacation from His Majesty's Army in Mesopotamia some forty years previously during the Great War of 1914-18. When we met, he was being squirreled away by my aunt in her flat in Neasden. I met him by chance when one of my visits coincided with one of his twice-weekly and very furtive forays to the tobacconist, off licence and bookmaker. Although my sightings of him were infrequent, he fascinated me and for many years my memories of him were an indelible benchmark for being old. As my birthdays pass, my fear of one day seeing Uncle Roger staring back at me from the mirror is thankfully diminishing and I am increasingly enthusiastic about getting older. I now believe it is really a very good idea. The real challenge is how to accumulate the birthdays and at the same time enjoy an increasingly greater quality of life; how to match the wisdom from experience with a fit, strong and capable mind and body.

As humans, we have many things in common with our fellow apes. There are, of course, a few obvious differences; most of us like to wear a few clothes and walk on our two hind legs for instance, and some of us are allowed to leave London Zoo without an ID card. Not so apparent is the difference in the way we humans age in comparison to our fellow primates. Humans are set apart by surviving long beyond the time when we cease to be fertile. There is an important evolutionary reason for this.

We take far longer to mature than our tree-climbing cousins, and our ability to survive long enough to nurture both children and grandchildren ensures the continuation and advancement of the earth's most complex and intelligent species. We live longer for a purpose, and as we get older the evolutionary expectation is that, with the exception of fertility, we should constantly improve our capabilities.

All of my experience, both personal and from working with others, suggests that there is no specific age at which we cease to be capable of further development. Continued development and longevity, however, are not accidents of fate; they require the investment of purpose, commitment and effort. All of the people I know who have immortality stand apart from their fellows because they deliberately nurture the following attributes:

- **Focus**; they know what they want from life and where they are going.
- **Positive outlook**; they believe in their dreams.
- **Mental capacity**; they are permanently seeking new challenges.
- **Self-respect**; they care about what they eat, their health and how they present themselves.
- **Capacity to enjoy life**; they believe in the pursuit of happiness. They believe in fun.

I have categorised these attributes into seven essential elements for achieving immortality. They are presented in order of priority and I recommend that you read, understand and master them in order. These essentials give you all the techniques you need to achieve your mental and physical best. Use them and you will never worry about the effects of ageing. Mental and physical wellbeing slows and often reverses the ageing process and, as if you needed an added bonus, this will be reflected in your appearance.

The first essential is to know where you are going and what you want in life. It is called *'Motivation and goals'*. A clear goal or vision of what you want in life is very motivating and will give you an invigorating sense of purpose.

The second essential is to make sure you have a positive outlook on life. It is called *'The power of being positive'*. It is vital to believe that you really can do what you want to do.

The third essential is about getting and keeping your brain in tip-top shape. It is called *'Flexing the mind'*. Not only will this help you to exploit your fitness and health to the maximum, but mental wellbeing plays a vital role in achieving health and fitness.

The fourth essential is called *'The importance of the body'*, and is all about what we have to do to achieve the fitness to walk-the-walk while talking-the-talk.

The fifth essential is called *'Eating for health'*, and gives information on how nutrition can assist super mental and physical health while still enabling you to enjoy what you eat. Eating is not only essential but also highly enjoyable. A few simple principles will heighten both the pleasure and the benefits.

The sixth essential is called *'Looking the part'*. It contains the fundamental information needed for a radiant and age-defying skin. How we look, and how we perceive that others see us, has a significant effect on our confidence. This confidence, or lack of it, has a significant impact on our social interactions with others.

The final essential is called *'Enjoy the sun, nature's free tonic'* and gives advice on how to safely benefit from the sun. I have included this because I encounter a lot of confusion about whether or not sunlight is harmful. The sun is essential for life, and exposure to it is vital for good health as well as a wonderful source of pleasure. The sun really does make immortality fun.

This book is dedicated to all those of my readers who want a little more out of life than finding their slippers in the morning. I hope I stimulate your mind with possibilities and that you find the information herein interesting and occasionally amusing. The contents of this book are not intended to be an alternative or substitute for medical opinion, and I recommend that everyone consults their medical practitioner before adopting a new diet or a new programme of exercise. For those of my readers who might feel disappointed, posthumously, that they did not manage to achieve eternal immortality, I have no hesitation in recommending my future publication, *'Immortality for Experts'*.

Acknowledgements

I would like to thank Simon and Liz for all of their help and encouragement in writing this book, and for their tireless efforts during the editing and formatting process. The assistance of my friend Paul to keep the content within the realms of science fact, rather than fiction, is also very much appreciated. I am also indebted to William, Georgia, Andy, David and Dave for all their help over the course of writing this book.

Any factual errors, poor grammar, and mizspelings that remain are completely my fault. I would also like to thank my wife, Sarah, and sister, Nina, for their patience and support, without which this book could not have been written.

Thanks are also due to Dave, Amanda and the team at Evade Black Belt School in Glossop, who transformed a fifty-six year old couch potato recovering from a broken hip into a sixty-two year old black belt ninja of the First Dan. They didn't allow my age to affect my perception of what I could do. For those of you that want to explore this exhilarating way of becoming really fit, I recommend that you look at their website at *www.evadeblackbeltschool.com*

Essential 1:
Motivation and goals

"What lies behind us and what lies before us are tiny matters compared to what lies within us."
– Ralph Waldo Emerson

A dog has a good life. He sleeps most of the time, probably dreaming of catching bunny rabbits. He doesn't have to worry about political correctness or membership of the European Union, he lets his owner do that. He doesn't have to worry where his next meal comes from, it somehow always does, and he has no ambitions about where he can go on holiday. He enjoys trips to the park with his mistress and will chase after balls and pieces of wood; if he's lucky he gets to romp around with other dogs, and on really special days maybe a bit of impromptu mating. World domination or saving the planet just doesn't interest him; all he wants is a rug by the fire, a pat on the head, and a well-chewed bone.

Humans are a little different. We need a reason for life that extends beyond satisfying our basic needs. If we didn't, we would still be strolling about the savanna, sniffing each other's armpits and scratching our heads. We have an innate sense of purpose that provides drive, direction and motivation beyond what is necessary to obtain the comfort of a pat on the head and a well-chewed bone. We all have that sense of purpose, even if we cannot all express what that purpose is or recognise what it means; it powered our ancestors' migration out of Africa to colonise the world, and to build a complex and advanced society. However, unless as individuals we can identify and describe it, we are unlikely to achieve and satisfy it. Motivation requires us to identify our sense of purpose and be consciously aware of how to fulfil it. Goals are the identified objectives of our sense of purpose.

Those of us who know both where we are going in life, and also want what we get when we get there, are fortunate. We will have purpose and energy; we will have motivation. Motivation is what gets us out of bed, smiling, on a Monday morning.

A fortunate few acquire their goals with little conscious effort. A teacher, a friend, a holiday, a film or a book is typical of the experiences that will trigger the all-consuming goals that will provide passion and meaning to our existence. However, for every person who has been lucky enough to have so easily and casually acquired the means of motivation there are thousands of others drifting through life waiting for Lady Luck to inspire them.

We all have a general awareness of what we seek in life. Tucked into our subconscious mind are the desires for health, happiness and abundance. Our subconscious mind holds these desires as abstract concepts against which it will evaluate all of our choices in life. To engage constructively with these desires they need to manifest themselves into specific forms that are real, tangible and achievable before they can become the goals that give us power and drive. We have two choices. We can either trust in chance and Lady Luck to prompt our subconscious with the 'eureka' moment, or we can use our conscious mind to test and explore those abstract concepts and to give them specific form. Goal setting requires the latter, making this choice is an essential part of taking control of your life.

I had a friend who was once possessed to pedal a very old, very rusty and very heavy bike up a very steep hill. Now that was a demonstration of pure motivation. However, for reasons known only to him, he carried on, over the hill, down the other side. In his determination to stay on his speeding and increasingly wobbly bike, he gripped the handlebars until his knuckles were white. That was pure fear. Near the bottom, as he flew over the handlebars when his front wheel came off, he extended his arms in front of him. That simple act of self-preservation was a great example of an incentive. I never asked him which part of the journey he enjoyed the most, but I expect it was the bit when he went uphill. Motivation always wins.

Being motivated makes life fun. Being motivated helps you achieve more. So let's make sure we're motivated!

• Are you doing it?
• Do you want to do it?
• Do you really want to do it?
• What's stopping you from doing it?

Because motivation is essential for success it is no accident that we begin our journey by discussing how to be truly motivated. So let's get started!

As we have discussed, motivation is the inner driving force that makes you want to do things and it will reward you by giving your inner-self pleasure from the act of doing. It is different to the external stimulus of incentives, which are often linked to achieving results and meeting targets.

When you are motivated, you perform a task for the intrinsic pleasure of doing it. This is not to say that incentives can't be used to help build motivation, but there is a risk that using incentives provides you with conflicting messages that might eventually have the opposite effect to that which was originally intended. For instance, if you promise yourself a bar of chocolate on completion of a three-mile jog, you may end up regarding the task in hand as a method of obtaining a bar of chocolate and, therefore, the jog becomes merely the price you have to pay. In this case, your motivation is obtaining the chocolate bar and the jog will become merely endured. This is a risky strategy as one day you will work out that it would be quicker, simpler and more efficient to just eat the chocolate and save a lot of time and effort in the middle. Contrast this with obtaining satisfaction with each and every step you take, each lungful of oxygen inside you, the air on your face, the feeling of physical empowerment and enjoying the wonderful buzz of adrenalin and endorphins.

So how do we get hold of this driving force? Motivating yourself to do something new sometimes requires a little bit of planning. So first of all you have to motivate yourself to motivate yourself! However, once you have done that, everything that follows is surprisingly easy. Before you can do this, you will have to know where you are going in life. Motivation and knowing your goals are immutably linked. You cannot be motivated unless you know where you are going and what you want to do, so in order to be motivated you need to discover your prime life goals.

"One of the greatest discoveries a man makes, one of his great surprises, is to find he can do what he was afraid he couldn't do." – Henry Ford

Discover your prime life goals

Do you want to be healthy?
Do you want to be wealthy?
Do you want to be happy?

I suspect that the answer for most people reading this book will be yes to all three of the above. However, if you are uncomfortable with declaring an enthusiasm for wealth, think about abundance; it is an ethically sympathetic alternative. Abundance in your life is when you don't have to worry about money. Wealth in your life is the same as having abundance, but with the added luxury of not worrying about being politically correct!

Acknowledging your desire for health, wealth and happiness is the first step in knowing what you want out of life. They are the prime needs of all humans and are incorporated into many national constitutions. Although they are universally aspired to, these goals will have different meanings for each of us, and you have to discover and understand what they mean to you as an individual. Your next task is to build a strong image of your life at a point in the future where you enjoy sufficient health, wealth and happiness to sustain contentment. Make the picture as complete as possible. This recognition of your desire for health, wealth and happiness is the first and most important stage in setting your goals.

Setting your prime life goals

To do this, you will need to set aside some time when you will be not disturbed. You will also need to find a peaceful space where you can be comfortable and relaxed. Remove as many distractions as possible – that means no TV, no radio and no mp3 player. Listening to R.E.M. or watching Aston Villa may satisfy uncertain needs for certain people, but they are not conducive to goal setting – no offence to Villa!

Step one:

Acknowledge the importance of health in your life. Imagine a life when you awake each morning bursting with energy, enjoying every breath of air, walking and playing with exuberance. Is this what you want? Form a picture in your mind of what health means to you.

Step two:

Acknowledge the importance of wealth in your life. Imagine a time when you have no financial concerns and you are able to easily afford all the things you want to do or have in life; holidays, cars, a nice house, university fees, charitable donations or helping friends and family. Is this what you want? Form a picture in your mind of what wealth, or abundance, means to you.

Step three:

Acknowledge the importance of happiness in your life. Imagine sharing the joy of living with your family and friends. Smiling and making others smile. Spending time and talking with those you like and love. Is this what you want? Form a picture in your mind of what happiness means to you.

Step four:

Recall all of your images of health, wealth and happiness and merge them into one comprehensive picture. Understand the relationships between health, wealth and happiness. Can you have one without the other? Is it possible to have complete happiness without health? Understand how each of the elements is dependent on the other two.

Step five:

Know your values. Values are those ethical principles by which you judge the actions of yourself and others, for instance, honesty, loyalty and so on. They define what we think is right or wrong and provide boundaries to what we do in life. We get our values from our experiences. More often than not, the majority of our values are those we obtained early in life from our parents and these values have been added to by our experiences at school, our religion, at work, from what we read, watch and listen to, by our friends and from life generally.

We will have different values for different areas of our life. These areas are often categorised as:

- Relationships
- Family
- Spirituality
- Health and fitness
- Personal development
- Career

Step six:

For each of the above categories, you need to make a list of your values and then explore and examine them until you fully understand what they mean to you. Be prepared for some surprises and be prepared for conflicts. For instance, if one of your values is to never tell a lie and another is loyalty, does that mean you would never tell a white lie, even when it was in the best interest of your closest friend to do so? Would you tell your neighbour's child that Santa doesn't exist? Would you never tell a loved one they looked good when you know your honest opinion would destroy their confidence? My experience of most values is that they are arbitrarily applied, and this is especially true of values that are a matter of fact, for example about lying or killing. Values that are more subjective such as loyalty and trust often are more consistent when you test them. Once you have examined your values, you should rank them in order of their importance to you. You should then test them as you would apply them to others and also as you would want others to apply them to you.

If, for instance, in the category of relationships you had listed the following values:

- Honesty
- Loyalty
- Confidentiality
- Compassion

You now need to think of an ethical dilemma that would challenge all four values.

If we take a hypothetical scenario where you had just been informed that your partner had been diagnosed with a life-threatening illness and that they had then specifically asked that your children not be told until more is known, what would you do if your child asked you about the health of their parent? Should you be honest and tell the child, thus breaking confidence and loyalty to your partner? Do you honour your confidentiality to your partner, but give a dishonest answer to your child? Do you show compassion to your partner by not telling your child or do you show compassion to your child?

Whatever you do, you will be unable to satisfy all of your values and one value will emerge as having a greater importance than the others. When you have finished this exercise, you should rewrite this list and make any consequent adjustments to how you rank your values in the order of importance.

You need to repeat this exercise at least one more time to check for conflicts and inconsistencies, such as whether the value of never telling a lie remains compatible with the value of compassion. Once you are sure of your values and their relative importance, you need to write them down.

Step seven:

Return to your image of health, wealth and happiness. You need to add substance to the picture. It is important that the image that you create is very strong; you must hear the sounds and smell the smells, as well as see it. Are there people in the image? What are they doing? What are you doing? The image must be so real that you must be in it and almost be able to touch it. You must see, feel and understand the pleasure it will give you.

There is a routine that will help you to build a complete picture. It requires having a question and answer conversation with yourself. Choose anything at random that you feel should be included in your picture of health, wealth and happiness. State what you have chosen, and then ask yourself: *'Which means?'*

When you ask this question of yourself, be prepared to think laterally and accept any answer that comes to mind. The purpose of these questions is to prompt the mind to develop a complete picture of your goals. There are no right or wrong answers, just more answers and a more detailed picture. Contemplate your answer, then once again ask *'Which means?'* and continue until you reach your general aspirations of health, wealth and happiness.

An example of this might go as follows:

- I'd like an old Jaguar E-Type roadster.
  (Now ask yourself: 'Which means?')
- I would need time to work on it and drive it.
  (Now ask yourself: 'Which means?')
- I would need a house with a large garage and barn.
  (Now ask yourself: 'Which means?')
- I need to buy a bigger house with outbuildings.
  (Now ask yourself: 'Which means?')
- I need to generate some money to spend on a bigger house.
  (Now ask yourself: 'Which means?')
- I need to have my own successful business.
  (Now ask yourself: 'Which means?')

And so on...

This conversation with yourself can be repeated as often as you like, and will provide different outcomes, each of which will add detail to the picture of your goals. For instance:

- I need to buy a bigger house with outbuildings.
  (Now ask yourself: 'Which means?')
- I'd like an old house.
  (Now ask yourself: 'Which means?')
- The house will be in the country.
  (Now ask yourself: 'Which means?')

- I will need to work from home to avoid commuting.
  (Now ask yourself: 'Which means?')
- I will need space for an office.
  (Now ask yourself: 'Which means?')

Constantly work on this goal image until it is highly detailed. Allow the threads of the questions and answers to take a random course.

In the first example above, I started by expressing a desire for a car, and the thread went via a larger house and a successful business. Eventually it will end at health, wealth and happiness. You need to work on these details until there are people in your picture together with sounds, movement, smells and emotions. The more complete the detail of this goal picture, the more effectively the picture will serve you as your prime goal that you will move towards with your life.

If you feel that the questioning has reached a dead end, go back a couple of questions and ask yourself 'how' or 'why' or 'what'. Do not worry if your line of thought goes off on a wild tangent. These wild tangents will provide valuable insights into the picture of your goals.

Your goal must always reflect the values you hold. Goals that reflect your values are ethical goals and will be more sustainable. It is good to periodically repeat the exercise on values. You are unlikely to achieve goals that conflict with your values.

Step eight:

Fix this goal to a time in the future; the time should be specific to the year and the month. It needs to balance realism with a certain amount of immediacy. If your goal is too far into the future, its pull will be too weak. However, if it is too immediate, you may consider it unrealistic. The majority of people will fix a goal somewhere between two and five years into the future, but everyone is different and it is important that the timescale works for you.

Step nine:

Make sure that your goal is achievable. Do you have the resources you need to achieve your goal? Do you need to obtain the resources, such as training, capital, and connections? Do you have the right attitude to achieve your goal?

Step ten:

Repeat steps four to nine as often as needed until you have a clear vision of where you are going. In other words, until the picture of your goal is so vivid, clear and detailed that it is almost real. A really intense vision will give you the strongest and most motivating goal. Your eventual goal will be:

- **Desirable**; It will reflect what you want in life. This is essential for a goal that will truly motivate you.

- **Achievable**; Do you have the resources to achieve it? Goals can be ambitious, unusual or innovatory, but they must always be realistic.

- **Compatible with your values and ethics**; You will never achieve goals that you think are ethically wrong. However, you will achieve goals that you think are ethically right; it makes your goals more desirable.

- **Compatible with the needs of your friends and family**; We are very social animals, and are unlikely to achieve and sustain goals that bring us into conflict with those we love and respect.

- **Fixed in a time frame**; We must know when we are going to fulfil our goals. The year and the month should be as much a part of your picture as the sights, sounds and people.

- **Sustainable**; This means that once you have achieved your goal, you will be able to remain in your fulfilling state of health, wealth and happiness for the foreseeable future. All prime life goals must be sustainable.

You may find it easier to perform the goal-setting exercises with the help of another person. This person will act purely as a facilitator. Their role will be to take notes of what you say and prompt you with the question, *'Which means?'* at the end of each statement. When a thread has reached an apparent end, they will revert to a previous answer and ask 'how' or 'why' or 'what' – as appropriate – to start a new thread.

The facilitator should not be judgmental, their purpose

is to keep the thread going wherever it takes you; his or her intervention should be kept to a minimum. It is important that the facilitator is a person you trust, and with whom you will not feel, in any way, self-conscious. The facilitator should help you to summarise all of the threads at the end of the session, and help you to test for desirability, achievability, compatibility with values, compatibility with the needs of friends, time frame and sustainability.

Now that you have set your prime life goals, we can use them as the motivating force to help you to achieve all of the individual milestone goals that eventually lead to where you want to be.

The value of clear and specific goals

Clear and specific goals have a value beyond being the source and inspiration for your motivation. They will facilitate success and achievement, and this is why they are advocated by all of the celebrity entrepreneurs in their self-help manuals. The reason, although simple, is powerful. If you know what you seek, you will always have a part of your subconscious mind that is looking out for opportunities that will help you to find and obtain it.

In every brain, at the core of the stem, is a vital component about the size of a juicy sultana that constantly monitors all of the information that the brain is receiving and processing. It is called the RAS (Reticular Activating System) and its purpose is to alert and focus the conscious mind on significant events. It enables us to walk and enjoy a conversation with friends, yet at the same time it will raise an alarm should we ever be in danger. It enables us to sit and read a newspaper in a busy and noisy airport lounge, yet hear our name called on the public address system. It separates all of the signals generated by the body while we walk and breathe while shopping, yet spot a friend in a crowd of strangers. Our RAS is always vigilant and, if we have a strong and clear image of what we seek, it will be forever watchful for opportunities to fulfil our goals while we enjoy the pleasures of our daily lives.

History has many famous examples of how our RAS has helped humanity to advance its knowledge. Archimedes had his 'Eureka' moment while enjoying a bath. His mind had been in deep contemplation about how to determine the metals that had been used in the making of a crown for his king, Hiero of Syracuse. To achieve this, he needed to know both the weight and the volume of the crown so that he could determine the density of the metal, and consequently the amount of gold used in its making. Ascertaining the weight was a simple matter of using scales, but determining the volume of the complex shape was the problem Archimedes took with him into his bath. As he lowered himself into the warm liquid, he noticed that the water level rose according to how much of his body was immersed, and he realised the displaced water was an indication of volume. He had found the answer. Legend has it that, in his excitement, he ran naked through the streets of Syracuse shouting *'Eureka! Eureka!'* – I have found it. This discovery enabled Archimedes to determine the density of the metals and, unfortunately for the king's goldsmith, also determine that silver had been substituted for some of the gold. There is no record of what happened to the goldsmith; however it is unlikely he shared the joy of Archimedes' important discovery.

In more recent times, this ability of our RAS to notice what we seek has led to the discovery of antibiotics. Sir Alexander Fleming, the Scottish biologist and pharmacologist, had been a Captain in the Royal Army Medical Corp during the carnage of the First World War. He had noticed how the use of antiseptics to fight infection in deeper wounds destroyed the body's immune cells, while still allowing the invading bacteria to breed, with devastating and often fatal consequences. Fleming witnessed many deaths from sepsis, and after the war dedicated himself to finding anti-bacterial agents that would be effective in the fight against infection. Although brilliant, he had a reputation as an untidy worker and typically, in 1928, before going on holiday, he placed all of his cultures of staphylococci bacteria on a bench in a corner of his laboratory. When he returned from holiday, he set about cleaning and tidying his laboratory, and noticed that one of the old cultures had become contaminated with a fungus, and the staphylococci bacteria had been destroyed. He immediately recognised the significance of the fungus in the petri dish, and set about refining it, thereby discovering penicillin.

"When I woke up just after dawn on September 28, 1928, I certainly didn't plan to revolutionise all medicine by discovering the world's first antibiotic, or bacteria killer", Fleming said, but that is what he had done; his ever-watchful RAS had alerted his mind to a possible solution to his problem. Fleming had discovered penicillin, and was awarded the Nobel Prize for Physiology or Medicine in 1945.

We might not wish to discover a new displacement theory or wonder-drug, but if our unconscious mind has a strong and clear image of what we seek it will, during all our waking hours, look out for the means for us to achieve our individual goals, whatever they are.

Task motivation

We enjoy most of our day-to-day activities and we look forward to doing a lot of them. There are, however, some jobs that just don't appeal. You know what they are, they're the ones you will find any and every excuse to delay doing. This normally doesn't present too much of a problem with small domestic tasks, but can create problems with less frequent tasks of greater importance.

For a lot of us, the annual tax return is a typical example. We know we have to do it. We have eight months in which to do it, but fifty per cent of us will delay doing it until the last possible moment, and many of us leave it to the last day. So many of us submit an online return in the final twenty-four hours that the HMRC website is subject to crashing, such is the volume of taxpayers logged on to the site. Every year we promise that next year we will submit our return early, but we know that each year we will continue to carry the dread of filing the return on our shoulders until the last possible moment. So why don't we do it early? It isn't that we can't do it, after all we do complete it, just very late! We also know the sense of relief and happiness we feel once we have done it. The reason we delay doing it is because we fail to motivate ourselves to do it.

When you have a task that you are reluctant to do, spend enough time putting it in context with your prime life goals. If it doesn't seem compatible with your goals, or it doesn't help you to achieve them, question whether you want or need to do it. If you do need or want to do it, then it has to be compatible with your prime life goals, but do not proceed until you understand why. Once you understand that completing a task is essential for achieving your goals, you will find it easier to do.

Secondly, you have to think of all the benefits, immediate and future, of performing your new task and then work on a strong image in your mind of how good you will feel when you are doing it, and how wonderful you will feel when you have completed it. Take the time to get this right. You must really want to do it. You must know how good you will feel when you have completed it. This might seem like the thinking man's alternative to procrastination, but once you master it you will find that it works.

Thirdly, you must introduce yourself to the activity in achievable steps, making sure that you have a strong image of the satisfaction and pleasure each step will give you. Each step you undertake should leave you wanting to do more. For instance, if you want to go jogging, don't start by forcing yourself through ten miles of mud and ice on a cold dark wet and windy day, unless of course that's what really turns you on. Start with a route within your capabilities that will let you enjoy each step, and, leave you with enough energy and enthusiasm to reflect on the pleasure that you will feel when you have completed it. If, at the end of your jog, you are left with a desire to do more, then you are on the way to building true and powerful motivation.

"A successful individual typically sets his next goal somewhat but not too much above his last achievement. In this way he steadily raises his level of aspiration."
– Kurt Lewin

Spend time each day reflecting on your achievements over the last twenty-four hours. Achievement is not about awarding subjective values of success or failure. Achievement is about activity and the effort you put into the activity. Think of the intrinsic pleasure the effort gave you and you will want to do more.

Make sure you reward yourself for achievement; the greatest reward is acknowledging your achievements and allowing yourself satisfaction. When you have done something well, spend time thinking about it. Think about the mental attitude that helped you to do something well and be pleased, very pleased. Do not dwell on events that haven't gone your way. Recognise any mistakes that you may have made, work out how you could have positively changed the outcome, and then move on.

Motivation is essential for immortality. Don't take it for granted, constantly work on it. Motivation comes from knowing your goals and really wanting them. If you are motivated, you will do more. The more you do, the more opportunities you will find and the more successful, interesting and enjoyable your life will be.

"A life spent making mistakes is not only more honourable, but more useful than a life spent doing nothing."
– George Bernard Shaw

The dos and don'ts of motivation

Do:

- Each morning, upon waking, contemplate and picture your prime life goals and relate them to the fulfilment of health, wealth and happiness.
- Each morning, put your tasks for the day into the context of your prime life goals. Before you proceed with your daily tasks, always be sure how they will enable you to achieve health, wealth and happiness.
- Each week, spend some time clarifying and intensifying the picture of your prime life goals.
- Each week, spend a little time prioritising your values. It is important to always be aware of your values.

- Set aside a little time at the end of each day to reflect on the satisfaction you have obtained from performing individual tasks during the day. Remember, it is not about success or failure, but the intrinsic pleasure of performing the task that is important.

Don't:

- Never undertake a task reluctantly. When you are reluctant to perform a task, you should spend enough time to put it into the context of your prime life goals.
- Never do anything until you are sure you want to do it.

Finally:
"Whatever you can do and dream you can do, begin it. Boldness has genius, power and magic."
– Johann von Goethe

Essential 2:
The power of being positive

"Enthusiasm is the yeast that makes your hopes shine to the stars. Enthusiasm is the sparkle in your eyes, the swing in your gait. The grip of your hand, the irresistible surge of will and energy to execute your ideas."
– Henry Ford

To gain immortality, we need to be positive. Being positive enables us to commit ourselves to life with enthusiasm. Being positive has great benefits.

I begin each day by making sure I am in a positive frame of mind, even more so when my life is particularly challenging. I know I am in control of my life when I feel positive. I deliberately avoid negative emotions; instead I look for happiness and focus on the future. When I do this, I can control stress and, in turn, this allows me to think with greater clarity and achieve more. It also enables me to be happy and enjoy each day. Life is too short to waste a single day on being miserable. Nora Ephron, the author of *'When Harry Met Sally'* and *'Silkwood'*, beautifully expressed this attitude in her address to graduates of Wellesley College in 1996, *"Above all,"* she said, *"be the heroine of your life, not the victim"*.

A positive outlook will bring a belief in your vision for the future, and this belief encourages persistence. Persistence is an essential element of the successful. More than 1,000 businesses refused to buy Colonel Sanders' chicken recipe before he found a buyer. After seven years of perseverance, at the age of seventy-five, he sold the company for $15 million. J.K. Rowling, in her 2008 address to Harvard graduates said, *"You might never fail on the scale I did. But it is impossible to live without failing at something, unless you live so cautiously that you might as well not have lived at all, in which case, you fail by default".* Twelve publishers rejected her manuscript until Bloomsbury Publishing agreed to publish it. In 2011, Forbes magazine, an influential American business publication, estimated J.K. Rowling's wealth to be approximately $1 billion.

So let's get positive!

- Can we do it?
- Will we do it?
- Come on, let's do it!

Do you still believe that one day you will fly into outer space, become prime minister, or discover lost continents?

"The future belongs to those who believe in the beauty of their dreams."

– Eleanor Roosevelt

One of the defining differences between the old and the young is belief in oneself. The younger we were, the more certain we were that one day, should we so choose, we could be the King of England or the President of the USA. Perhaps even both, after all the choice was endless. We gave our imagination full rein – or should that be reign – without any consideration of futility.

When we were young, everything was possible and our ambition was driven by the direction in which we happened to be looking. As we age, we restrict our choice of actions to those that we perceive we can do, and consequently for most of us the result is that our choice of actions becomes smaller and smaller.

It is a vicious cycle. The narrower our comfort zone, the less we expose ourselves to the chance of new experiences until eventually our lives are restricted to a small collection of activities and behaviours. At this stage, physical and mental deterioration is the inevitable consequence, and the Grim Reaper squints his eye as he looks for your name on his schedule.

Having a positive outlook is vital for a youthful life. It is almost impossible to maintain a spring in your step when you believe you are walking to despair and doom, at least for any worthwhile period of time. It's difficult to look forward to a life of new challenges if you anticipate catastrophe instead of exciting experiences. If you are positive, you will be able to hope, and with hope comes anticipation and a belief in the future. If you believe in the future, you have retained one of the wonderful gifts of youth.

The consequences of having a negative outlook are self-fulfillingly grim. Apart from having a more-than-good chance of becoming a stereotypical miserable grump leading a life of gloom, you run a high risk of being cynical. Not to mention bitter and undoubtedly twisted, and probably paranoid too! Your friends will melt away, and without doubt you will enter the nightmare of your dotage that matches your worst fears.

However, if you insist on being miserable as a lifestyle choice then the good news for you is that current research indicates that people who do not have a positive outlook tend to live an average of five years less, and in poorer health. Unhappy people tend to be stressed, and that stress is accompanied by increased cortisol production, a higher heart rate and higher levels of blood sugar and immunosuppression – a weakening of the body's immune system.

There has been a lot of research in the last two decades into the connection between feeling positive and happy and being in good health. In a 2005 study of 216 British civil servants, the happiest civil servants had the lowest level of the stress hormone cortisol and plasma fibrinogen, an indicator of inflammation that is associated with heart disease[1].

Another study, completed in 2011 by epidemiologists at University College London, surveyed over three thousand people aged between fifty-two and seventy-nine who were assessed for happiness, contentment, worry and fear[2]. This large sample was divided into three groups according to their scores and, at the end of five years, their mortality was recorded. The mortality rate of the most positive group over the five years was half that of the most negative group, leading them to suggest that happiness is good for health.

There has been a significant amount of research into the health benefits of being positive, and it continues to increase as the evidence mounts. In 2012, a team at the Harvard School of Public Health in Boston, Massachusetts, completed a review of 200 separate research studies that looked at psychological wellbeing and cardiovascular health, especially coronary heart disease and strokes. Their conclusion was that a positive outlook had a substantial beneficial effect on health. Julia Boehm, the lead author of the study, gave the following summary: *"The absence of the negative is not the same as the presence of the positive. We found that factors such as optimism, life satisfaction and happiness are associated with reduced risk of cardiovascular disease regardless of such factors as a person's age, socio-economic status, smoking status or body weight. For example, the most optimistic individuals had an approximately fifty per cent reduced risk of experiencing an initial cardiovascular event compared with their less optimistic peers."*

A significant benefit of being positive is that you will be more resistant to stress and, as a consequence, you will be more likely to avoid overproduction of the hormone cortisol. This hormone is critical as it enables the body to cope with stress. However, an excess of cortisol is very damaging, not only to the heart and body as we have seen above, but also to the brain. The brain has neurons that are very sensitive to an excess of the hormone.

Cortisol is also increasingly linked to the ageing process, and an excess is associated with lower levels of testosterone, muscle wasting, bone loss, thinning skin, poor recovery from wounds and a build-up of abdominal fat[3]. One of the most immediate and apparent symptoms of excess cortisol is extreme fatigue.

Fortunately, there are five easy ways that you can influence your cortisol production: diet, moderate exercise, sleep, mental happiness and relaxation, all of which we discuss in this book. Being positive is an essential element of mental health and happiness, and consequently an important element in the strategy to reduce cortisol levels. This, in itself, should go a long way to motivate you to persevere with being positive.

"To accomplish great things, we must not only act, but also dream; not only plan, but also believe."
– Anatole France

Being positive is something you can influence. Although some research indicates that a positive or negative outlook is significantly affected by genetics, the same research shows it is almost equally affected by your activities. Not only can you affect whether or not you are positive or negative, but also how positive you are. The following tasks are essential to having a positive outlook.

Having goals

I discussed goal setting a little in the previous chapter on motivation. Now is the time to put a bit of flesh on the goals you set earlier. We had set a goal in our mind where we enjoyed health, wealth and happiness. Go back to that image and build up the detail.

• Who is there with you?
• Are they happy?
• Where are you?
• What have you just done?
• What are you doing?
• What are you about to do?
• What can you hear?
• What can you smell?
• What can you touch?

This image should be set at a definite and not too distant point in the future. This is an image that you must constantly work on and visit daily. A very strong image of your goals will help you in many ways, and this includes maintaining a positive outlook. Whenever you feel negative thoughts or emotions taking hold, bring back that image of your goals and remind yourself of the bigger picture of where you are going. The more complete and thorough the image of your goals, the more effective it will be in keeping you in a positive frame of mind.

Move towards your goals. We are attracted to what we want, and are repelled by what we fear and dislike. The power of attraction is far more powerful and enduring than fear and dislike. Attraction becomes greater the closer we get to what we want, whereas repulsion diminishes the further away we are from what we dislike and fear.

An example a lot of us will identify with is losing weight. Some us will lose weight because we consider ourselves too heavy, some of us decide we want to be a target weight. I expect most of those who diet do it because they think they are too heavy are likely to be perpetually dieting. This is because the further away you get from the despised weight, the less you feel the need to diet, and once again one more doughnut slips through the guilt defences. However, for those that want to achieve a target weight, the nearer to the target you get, the more inspired and committed you become. Success will always follow if you move towards where you want to be. The closer you get to your goals, the more attainable they become and the happier you will be.

Positive review of events

Whenever you think you have received a setback, review every aspect of the events in question. Look for lessons that you have learnt, and consider how these lessons will make you more successful in the future. Also, look for any positive outcomes from the events however incidental. These might not have been the primary objective of your activities, but everything positive has a benefit and every benefit leaves you better off. These positive outcomes could be knowing someone better, understanding processes, finding shortcuts or noticing new things. The possibilities are endless, so open your mind and explore them.

Stop worrying

Let other people do the worrying. Worrying is the biggest waste of time in the universe so, if you want to move on, you must replace it with thinking of how you will make your life better, this is far more productive. This is not to say that you must avoid facing up to events that make you uncomfortable, but your responsibility to yourself is to deal with those events as efficiently as possible so that you can move on and achieve your goals.

I would expect that most of us can look back to a time in our teenage years when we felt that the end of the world was more certain than our next meal. A time when tomorrow was scarcely worth waking up to, and somehow we were locked into an eternity of life being worse than the death of a thousand cuts. Despite this, many years later, you are now reading this book having experienced at least one or two gloriously happy moments during the interval.

If you reflect on all the worrying you once did, you will hopefully appreciate that not only was it a complete waste of time, but you would have been a lot happier a lot sooner had you moved on to your future with a bit more urgency. Worrying achieves nothing, so remove it from your life.

Get good quality sleep

Sleep on it. Good sleep is good for the mood, so make sure you get enough. Sleep has the added benefit of allowing your unconscious mind to digest all of the information it has acquired while you have been awake.

However, good sleep won't accidentally happen. It is important to go to sleep in the right frame of mind. If you go to bed with all of your worries churning through your mind, then there will be two counterproductive tendencies. The first is that you probably won't get much sleep as you lie awake worrying. The second is that your subconscious mind will be processing all of the things in your day that are negative rather than looking for positive outcomes.

When you go to bed, focus on comfortable positive thoughts.

Preferably take your mind to a place where you want your goals to lead you. If you do this, you are far more likely to wake up refreshed and energised and you will be surprised at how likely you are to find new solutions to any problems and challenges that face you. There is an old adage that problems are best solved by sleeping on them. There is truth in it, and sleep is an essential requirement for immortality. In the next chapter, *'Flexing your mind'*, a fuller explanation of sleep is given, together with a description on how your circadian clock affects your body.

Get enough sunlight

Get some early morning sun. One of the ways your body calibrates itself is to use ultraviolet radiation to stimulate the production of serotonin and melatonin, two substances that, among other things, enhance your mood. The ultraviolet radiation has to be detected by the eyes, so leave the sunglasses in your pocket; unless of course the glasses happen to be Ray Bans and you happen to be Italian, in which case you may stick them on top of your head.

Later, at the end of the book, there is a chapter on safety in the sun. All the many benefits of sunlight are explained, and there is good advice on how to get the benefits while avoiding the risks.

Eat the right foods

Food is a wonderful thing. For most of us, eating can be a great source of pleasure and many of us have special foods, usually involving chocolate and sugar, that are always certain to move our mind into a happy heaven. We are probably less aware of the effect that deficiencies in our diet have on our mood.

Research into food and mood is gathering pace as the shortcomings of relying on a purely medical approach, not least the expense, is providing a strong incentive to find ways of managing mood disorders without medical intervention. The most promising of the research has been focused on EPA (Eicosapentaenoic acid), a polyunsaturated fatty acid that is found in fish oil or oily fish such as salmon, mackerel and sardines. These fish oils are often referred to as essential fatty acids (EFA) or omega-3 acids, however it is worth noting that not all EFAs contain EPA and that fish oil remains the richest source. The positive effect of EPA in countering anxiety and depression is increasingly established and documented[4].

It isn't just fish oil that brings these benefits. Vegetables high in antioxidants have also been shown to have benefits, and even much-maligned red meat plays an important role[5].

A recent study of 1,000 Australian women, conducted by the Deakin University in Victoria, Australia, revealed a strong connection between eating red meat and reducing depression and anxiety disorders[6]. However, the conclusion of the research was that the benefits were specific to eating about 70 grams – about the size of burger – of grass-fed beef and lamb, and not from eating other meats such as chicken or pork. This is good news for all those steak lovers who are dispirited about constant warnings about the perils of red meat. I suspect that it is also excellent news to wombats, koala bears, kangaroos and all of the other alternative sources of red meat that occasionally become Sunday lunch on an Australian barbecue.

The benefits of a varied diet including fish and meat are more fully explained in *Essential 5: 'Eating for health'*.

Positive language

Use the right language: positive language. Your mood is largely controlled by your subconscious mind and this makes it very difficult to change on demand. This is something I suspect most of us occasionally attempt to do and fail.

What we can do is train our subconscious mind so that it tends towards positive thoughts and emotions. The way we achieve this is with the language we use. The language we use, either internally or when talking to others, is something we control with our conscious thoughts. If we use positive and definite language then, in time, the personality of our subconscious will become positive and definite.

Avoid negatives

You should abandon as many negative expressions as is possible. Avoid saying 'I can't' but say what you need to do instead. If you are asked to do something you don't do, then say you don't do it, if you haven't got time to do it, then say you haven't got time to do it. There is nothing that you cannot do if you put enough effort into it, so never say you can't do something. Never say you will try, because 'try' is just a way of saying you won't without taking responsibility for saying you won't. Take the decision to always phrase what you will do as a positive 'I will do'.

It is equally important to avoid making general assumptions that are negative, especially assumptions that are about other people. How often have you heard the expression 'everybody hates me' or 'the world is against me'. A little thought about such statements reveals that they cannot possibly be true and that the assumptions are baseless – even Attila the Hun had friends! However, making such statements will, in time, have a negative effect on your subconscious personality. Persevere with your decision to think positively and definitely. The good news is that once you have adopted the habit of talking positively, whether to yourself or others, you will find your personality and attitude will in time become positive too.

Laughter

Laughter is important. We owe the word 'laugh' to the Germans, as it is derived from the Old High German *'hlahhan'*. We should also thank the Germans for taking it sufficiently seriously that, at a school in the northern quarter of Berlin, you can learn to laugh. Here you can see potentially happy Germans running around shouting 'ho, ho, ho' and 'ha, ha, ha' under the tutelage of Mirthmeister Susanne Maier – motto "Fake it until you make it" – a laughter therapist.

Laughter is not only good exercise for the lungs, it also releases endorphins that make you feel good. Try to laugh as early in the day as possible, as it sets you up in the right mood. If you can't find anything to make you laugh, just imagine you are in a school in the northern quarter of Berlin, and laugh. If this doesn't work try laughing with a German accent! This is best done standing up, so don't leave it until you're driving in a car – even a German car – and definitely don't wait until you're standing on the train.

Remember that happiness is a matter of the right chemicals in the brain. Laughter is one of many effective ways that you can legally get those chemicals working for you.

Triggers

Everybody has a trigger that will make them feel happy, and feeling happy is the first step to feeling positive. Triggers vary enormously, but frequently involve locations, people, clothes, food and music. It pays to identify these triggers so that you can use them to feel good either about yourself or about events.

There is a caution to using foods though, as this could lead to weight problems and eventually that would have a negative effect. The best triggers are locations, clothes and music as these are all things you can easily access. There is a plus side to using these triggers too, as each time you use them they have a stronger effect.

The really great thing about triggers is that once you have identified them you can incorporate them into your lifestyle. If you know that certain clothes make you feel good, always wear them. Fill your ears with the music that lifts your mood and surround yourself with the people that stimulate your soul. Why wait until you are miserable?

If you are willing to persevere, you can also create a type of physical trigger, which is called an anchor. For this, you have to choose an area of the body that is both accessible and capable of being stimulated in a discreet manner, such as the ear lobe or part of the little finger. Your next task is to get yourself into the required state of happiness. This you can do by either recalling vivid memories of very happy events or by using one of the triggers we have already discussed. You will find the intensity of happiness comes in waves and you will need to anticipate when the feeling will be at its greatest. When the state of happiness is about to peak, you should stimulate – usually by pressing or squeezing – the anchor, and continue to stimulate until the peak starts to subside. This exercise should be repeated about six times, and then tested and repeated again until you are able to recall the desired intensity of happiness.

This technique can be used on most emotional states, such as enthusiasm, confidence, calm and so on. In order for the anchor to be long-lasting, it is important to choose an anchor that is unlikely to be accidently stimulated.

Positive posture

When boxers train, they are told to stand in a way that makes themselves look, and feel, like a boxer. One purpose is to scare their opponent to death, which doesn't often happen. The other purpose is to get them into a fighter's mind-set, and this always happens. If you look the part, you will find it easier to play the part, and you should apply this to being positive. There is a causal relationship between mental and physical posture. Your physical stance will affect your mental stance, and vice versa. So stand tall, shoulders back, smile and walk with confidence. If you are unused to doing this, then start by wearing the clothes that you like the most, stand in front of a mirror, breathe deeply using the stomach, stand tall and marvel at how good you look. Breathe in deeply, and smile!

There has been fascinating research on the effect that your posture has on your mood. Charles Darwin is famous for his work on evolution, but in 1872 he also published a book about the implications of facial expressions, called 'The Expression of Emotions in Man and Animals'. This work eventually evolved into the 'Facial Feedback Hypothesis', which states that facial movement can influence emotional experience.

More recent research has broadened the implications of this research. In 2010, a team at Columbia University examined the psychological and behavioural effects of posturing by taking a group of men and women and getting them to assume either high or low power postures[7]. Not only did the high power group have a higher propensity to take risk, but saliva tests also revealed an increase in testosterone levels. Testosterone is a hormone associated with dominance and power. The low power group revealed increased levels of cortisol in their saliva. Cortisol is a hormone that is linked to stress, triggered by powerlessness and anxiety, and a lower incidence of risk-taking. The effect of posture goes beyond the psychological, and has a demonstrable physiological effect as well.

Posture has also been recently shown to have a remarkable effect on creativity. In a study at North Dakota State University, psychologist Michael Robinson randomly assigned several hundred undergraduates into two groups. He gave the following instruction to one of the groups: *"You are seven years old. School is cancelled, and you have the entire day to yourself. What would you do? Where would you go? Who would you see?"* The other group was given the same instructions, but with the first sentence omitted: *"School is cancelled, and you have the entire day to yourself. What would you do? Where would you go? Who would you see?"* After writing on this topic for a short period, they were given a set of tasks to test their creativity. The group that had imagined themselves as seven-year olds came up with twice as many ideas than the other group. This is compelling evidence that posture is a powerful tool for achieving your goals.

For me the evidence is clear; being positive brings huge benefits to your mental and physical health. You can choose whether you want to be positive. If you choose to be positive, act positive and you will be positive.

"Many of life's failures are people who did not realise how close they were to success when they gave up."
– Thomas A. Edison

The dos and don'ts of being positive

Do:

- Ensure that you start the day in a happy and positive frame of mind. If necessary, force yourself to smile and laugh. If you are still struggling, try whistling, it always works. My father had a dog that whistled; it couldn't remember any tunes, but it always seemed very happy.

- Think about all of the things you have done in the last five days. These are all achievements and successes, however small they may seem. Well done.

- Think about how you can make someone happy today.

- Think about something that has happened to you recently that has made you happy.

- Wear clothes that you like and that also give you confidence.

- Adopt a positive posture. Stand upright in a confident pose, smile and breathe deeply.

- Listen to music that lifts your mood.

- Only use positive language, in both speech and thoughts.

- Say 'I can' if you are able to do something. Say 'I will' if you want to do it. You can achieve anything you want to if you believe in yourself.

- Seek out people, events and other things that make you feel happy and positive.

- Develop triggers that you can use to make yourself positive and happy.

Don't:

- Never worry. Life is too short, even if you adopt all seven essentials into your lifestyle. Contemplate how good life will be when a problem is solved. Think about something that you enjoy. Never, ever worry. It is a waste of time and interferes with the important task of creating solutions. It never accomplishes anything.

- Don't communicate with negative people. If this is unavoidable, communicate by writing. Send them all of your bad news, it will make them happy. Use second class post and give them someone else's address for the reply.

- Never say you will 'try'. You will always fail if you try. Make a decision whether or not you are going to do something. If you decide to do something, you will do it!
- Don't use negative language. If you say 'you can't', you never will.

Essential 3:
Flexing the mind

To achieve immortality, we need a keen brain that can understand, reason and plan.

Whenever I am in Manchester, I like to find time to visit my favourite library, The Portico, and have lunch. Its history makes it a special place. Muriel the cook brings your meal to you in the little reading room at the back; a wonderful room of bookshelves, worn leather armchairs and complete calm. The Portico has had many famous members, among them William Gaskell, Sir Robert Peel and John Dalton. It was here that Dr Roget, the first secretary of the Portico, compiled his famous thesaurus; a task that he started when he was sixty-one and finished when he was seventy-three.

Roget was not the only person to make a significant intellectual contribution in later life. Caspar Wessel, the almost unknown Danish mathematician, was the first person to describe the geometrical interpretation of complex numbers in the complex plane. He published his fundamental paper *'Om directionens analytiske betegning'* in 1799 at the age of fifty-four. Unfortunately, he published in Danish, and his work went unnoticed until it was republished in French in 1899. In the field of music, Cesar Franck composed his *'Symphony No.1 in D'* at the age of at fifty-six, and Leos Janacek wrote *'Jenufa'* in 1904, at the age of fifty. In the field of literature, Raymond Chandler published his best seller *'The Big Sleep'* at the age of fifty-one, and Richard Adams published his first novel *'Watership Down'* when he was in his fifties. However, the prize for never stopping has to go to Nirad Chaudhuri, who published his final work *'Three Horsemen of the New Apocalypse'* at the age of one hundred, two years before his death in 1999.

So now we know that age is no barrier to mental brilliance, let us sharpen our minds.

- Can you think?
- Are you thinking?
- What are you thinking?

"When I was a boy of fourteen, my father was so ignorant I could hardly stand to have the old man around. But when I got to be twenty-one, I was astonished at how much the old man had learned in seven years."
– Mark Twain

There is a popular modern proverb that says 'age and treachery will always overcome youth and skill'. I find this thought very reassuring, and I am rather thankful that getting older may bring certain competitive advantages. However, treachery isn't the only advantage that I have, which is fortunate because despite my years and carefully hidden ambition, treachery is something that I have yet to completely master. What I do have, in common with everyone else who accumulates the years, is an increasing wealth of experience. Some of this experience is about how to achieve things happily, easily and successfully. Most of it, however, is about the apparently random, and totally unexpected, outcomes that often follow meticulous planning and obsessive execution.

Fortunately, all experience is good, and all experience can be used to guide us to a more fulfilling life. Having said this, experience is but a library in the mind. If you never use it, you will never benefit from it. To use it you need recall and reasoning, you need to learn from it and adapt it to your current circumstances. To use it well you will require a razor sharp intellect and all the rest of your cognitive capabilities in full working order, and this is only possible with a bit of well-planned effort.

Use it or lose it

The clever and capable brain is not an accident; it is a deliberate choice that requires commitment and a moderate amount of hard work.

We live in a society where the expected fruit of our labours is relaxation that too often involves sedating our brains with effortless entertainment. We indulge for pleasure in activities that allow our cognitive powers to decay in a state of self-induced oblivion. Not only does the brain require exercise to keep it functioning, like your body it will also continue to develop and improve if you exercise it correctly. If you neglect your precious brain it will fade away without you knowing.

Your brain requires challenging exercise, and the evidence to confirm this is compelling. In 2010, a team of French and British doctors published a report that concluded that the number of dementia sufferers could be reduced by 40 per cent[8]. Some of this effect was due to diet, but the report concluded that almost half of the improvement would be achieved by involvement in education, especially literacy. Among the recommended activities was continuing in education and reading and writing more. The report also predicted that, if no action is taken, around one million people will suffer from dementia by 2015. This study is one of many.

In 2009, researchers at the Institute of Psychiatry at King's College, London analysed data from 1,320 dementia sufferers. They found that, for the majority of men continuing to work on late in life, the brain was kept healthy enough to stop dementia taking hold. There are many similar reports and their message is clear; if you want a brain that works, you have got to work it hard. Mental exercise isn't the only factor; physical exercise, diet and lifestyle play equally important roles, but it's mainly mental exercise that we are considering in this chapter.

"Anyone who stops learning is old, whether at twenty or eighty. Anyone who keeps learning stays young. The greatest thing in life is to keep your mind young."
– Henry Ford

The secret of success is to convince your grey matter that thinking is fun, and fortunately there is a fantastic variety of ways to achieve this. The first step, however, is to realise that enhancing and maintaining your mental capabilities is the most important task in your life, and is consequently the one task you must always find time for. When you have set your prime goals in life, you will realise how essential the capacity for complex and reasoned thought is in achieving those goals. This realisation will assist in your motivation to exercise your mind which, in turn, will reward you with satisfaction and pleasure – and consequently further motivation – from the tasks of thinking, learning and problem solving. To a certain extent, you have to learn how to learn and at the same time associate the whole process with satisfaction and pleasure. Once you have started to achieve this, you will discover that exercising your brain gathers self-motivating momentum.

The human brain is truly incredible. It is made up of neurons or nerve cells of which there are approximately 100 billion; in other words, you have thirteen times more neurons in your brain than there are people on this earth. On the basis of body size, our brain is the biggest of all the primates and this increase is significantly due to the enhanced size of our cerebral cortex, the part that is responsible for planning, reasoning, language and abstract thought. Our brains are expensive, about one-fifth of the energy used by the body is consumed by the brain, more than any other organ. It also requires one-fifth of the oxygen and requires fifteen per cent of the cardiac output from the heart. Do not be surprised if thinking makes you both tired and hungry!

Learning how to learn

"Nothing is particularly hard if you divide it into small jobs."
– Henry Ford

Learning how to learn is best done in small stages. It is a process of undertaking a task until performing the task provides intrinsic pleasure and satisfaction. If you have already performed the task before and enjoyed doing it, then carry on doing it. However, the following technique of learning how to learn is recommended for tasks that you haven't performed before.

You need to start by breaking the task down into as many mini-tasks as possible so that each mini-task is a determinable process with an identifiable start and end. When you begin to perform one of these mini-tasks, it should be performed without any regard to the outcome because your initial purpose is to learn to enjoy the actual process.

For instance, if you want to learn how to do quadratic equations – I'm assuming in this instance you may have chosen to forget your entire knowledge of algebra – you should start by solving simple 'x,y' equations, and continue with them until the actual process brings you pleasure and satisfaction. Only when this has been achieved should you include a successful outcome in your criteria for pleasure and satisfaction. Once you can perform the first mini-task to your satisfaction, continue with the next mini-task and, when that has been successfully learnt, join the first two mini-tasks together. Remember that for the purpose of learning how to learn, the pleasure and satisfaction of doing is of greater value than the result.

New challenges

One of the most obvious ways of stretching and developing the mind is commencing new pursuits. Finding a new pursuit should be done on a regular basis – it should become a pursuit in itself. There three major benefits from a new pursuit.

The first is that by undertaking something new, you are expanding the scope of your horizons and with that you will bring into your life an exponential increase in new ideas and cognitive challenges. You will be going against a trend of ageing where your range of activities would normally become more restricted as you become older. This benefit is enhanced because a new pursuit will undoubtedly cause you to come into contact with new people and this, in turn, will expose you to yet more new ideas and experiences. These new experiences will become increasingly unpredictable and random as your horizons become broader. This not only makes for a truly interesting life, but is also exceptionally stimulating for your mind.

The second benefit is that new pursuits require the learning of new techniques and knowledge, which is excellent exercise for the brain. In fact, learning a new pursuit normally involves quite a comprehensive workout for the old grey matter. One aspect will be the acquisition, storage and retrieval of new information, another aspect will be the understanding and solving of new problems. If the pursuit involves physical activity, multiple lobes of the cerebral cortex will be used mastering new motor skills, including mind-body coordination and so, apart from the physical benefits to the body, it is a total mental workout.

For a real mental challenge, learn how to play a musical instrument or learn a new language. Learning a new musical instrument doesn't have to be particularly expensive, as many music shops will rent out instruments to students – even to students with an over-sixties bus pass! If renting isn't your cup of tea, cheap but playable musical instruments are increasingly available from the new Asian economies, such as China. This may have an added advantage if the instructions are in Chinese, as you will be provided with the additional opportunity of learning a new language. If you are really lucky, the instructions will have been translated into that unique version of the English language known only to Chinese technical translators, and understood by no-one. In this event, not only will you be learning a musical instrument and a foreign language, but you will also, by the time you have reached the bottom of the first page of the instruction manual, have become expert at code-breaking.

The third benefit is that everything new that you learn or discover may provide that vital step to achieving your goals. Goals are, by definition, aspired achievements set in the future. The fact that you have not yet achieved them is because all of the actions and resources required for their achievement are not yet known, understood or available to you.

Puzzles for playtime

On a more casual basis, solving puzzles and crosswords is a great method of improving computational and reasoning skills. By choosing a good variety of puzzles, you can exercise almost all of the parts of the cerebral cortex, as well as improving memory retention and recall. Variety is also the spice of life, so your enjoyment will increase as you extend the range of your mental challenges. Most types of puzzles are readily available, either on the Internet, as mobile phone applications or in daily newspapers. They have the great advantage of convenience as they require very little in the way of prior planning and organisation, and are a great way to casually utilise small packets of time. Below are some puzzles worth considering.

Tangrams

Tangrams are dissection or tiling puzzles that involve making geometric images from seven defined flat shapes. They are great way to develop spatial awareness, and involve a lot of abstract thought. Spatial awareness is essential for creating solutions to complex problems, such as those that may be found in engineering, architecture and mathematics. Tangrams have a great advantage in that a very useable puzzle will fit into an area no greater than the size of a CD case. This little puzzle has an almost infinite life; it is estimated that there are over 6,500 possible configurations for the seven pieces – and more are being created.

Sudoku

Although they involve numbers, the solving of sudokus only minimally involves mathematics. A sudoku is a logic-based number placement puzzle that has nine 3 by 3 grids. They require the development of a methodical approach to problem solving, and are a great way to exercise the lobes in the cortex that deal with planning and abstract thought. They also have the advantage of being very available and can be found in most daily newspapers. There are now a lot of computerised sudoku games freely available, either on the Internet or as applications for mobile phones.

The number of possible solutions for these puzzles is popularly quoted as 6,670,903,752,021,072,936,960, which is probably best expressed as 6.67×10^{21}. However you express the number, it is a lot and probably enough for most lifetimes, but unfortunately it is insufficient for the dedicated immortal. Quite a few sudokus now have a target time for completion, but my advice is that the target time serves very little purpose, unless of course doing them all before you die is on your Bucket List. The speed at which you will solve a sudoku will depend on how fresh or tired your mind is. If you tackle a sudoku when you are tired, you are highly likely to exceed the target time and perhaps regard your efforts as somehow consequentially failing. However, I would reason that completing a sudoku when the brain is tired is a great achievement, regardless of the time taken.

Crosswords

Fifteen years ago, crosswords were not only the most popular puzzle, but frequently the only puzzle published in daily newspapers. Now they make only a small contribution to the puzzle pages found in all of the dailies. Despite this, they are an exceptionally good form of mental exercise.

At their simplest level, crosswords are simply a test of general knowledge, synonyms and word meanings, yet even at this level they are excellent at developing powers of sorting, matching and retrieving information. More complex crosswords are called cryptic crosswords and they involve the creation of words from clues. These cryptic crosswords use all of the same parts of the brain as the simpler crosswords, but they also develop powers of reasoning and abstract conceptualisation.

Legend has it that, at one time, entry to the Secret Service was dependant to a certain extent on being able to complete the cryptic crossword in the Daily Telegraph, a legend probably based on a true story concerning the breaking of the German Enigma code during the Second World War. During those dark days, Britain was almost entirely dependent on supplies being sent across the Atlantic by boat, and this fragile lifeline was constantly threatened by the deadly U-Boats. Over 3,500 merchant vessels were sunk and the survival of the convoys hung upon the ability to crack the Enigma code at Bletchley Park, the historic site of the secret British code-breaking operation, and the birthplace of the modern computer. There was an urgent need for people who had the particular mental agility to become cryptologists, and to help quickly find the right candidates, a particularly challenging crossword competition was held in the Telegraph. As history shows, the competition was a success, and the Battle of the Atlantic was won[9].

All puzzles are worth doing. There is merit in doing as many puzzles as possible, rather than focusing on trying to do a few puzzles well. From the point of view of developing your cognitive powers, the benefit is in the doing rather than the result or whether you perform comparatively better than others. My advice is to do any puzzle you can get your hands on, regardless of how simple or complex it is; however, the more effort it involves, the better.

Competitive games

Competitive games have diminished in popularity in the last two decades, significantly as a result of the advances in computerised gaming. Playing computer games can benefit cognitive ability, especially in the areas of making very quick calculations and spatial awareness. Very few computer games however, can stimulate as many areas of the brain as the competitive games of chess or even bridge. Chess, for instance, requires complex planning many moves in advance, assessing potential threats, calculating risks and developing strategies. It develops the ability for deep reasoning and abstract conceptualisation to deal with the multiple and unpredictable outcomes of playing a human adversary. Because of the human involvement, these games involve complex social skills such as posture and bluff – not to mention a dash of treachery – as well as an opportunity to assess your opponent.

Gamesmanship is fun, and requires a great deal of skill and practice to do it well. Competitive games are normally doubly motivating because the motivation that comes from the intrinsic enjoyment of the game is enhanced by the motivation to win. When the motivational force is very strong, it is likely that the brain is stretched beyond its normal limits and, because of this, competitive games are a great way to expand cognitive capacity.

Using the brain, not the calculator

Calculators are wonderful things. You can now calculate seven-figure sums precise to ten decimal places as fast as your fingers can enter the numbers. The time saved when calculating the square root of two, precise to nine decimal places, is considerable. Unfortunately, each time you use a calculator, your brain will lose some of its processing power until eventually you will be unable to perform even the simplest of mental arithmetic.

The good news, however, is that this atrophy of the brain is significantly reversible; if you start using your brain again, you will find that it will become increasing capable of complex calculations. Most calculations that we need to do in our everyday life require accuracy rather than precision. For instance, when you check your supermarket bill for accuracy, it is important to be able to quickly estimate your bill within the price of the cheapest article, and subsequently totalling the bill to the nearest penny is an irrelevant precision.

The next time you reach for a calculator, stop yourself and give your brain a chance – the more you allow your brain to make the calculations, the more calculations the brain will want to do. An even greater benefit is that the brain will start to calculate in the subconscious, giving you a superb numerical intuition that will reward you many times over in enhanced speed of decision-making.

Staying curious

We are all curious, but too many of us regard curiosity as an unwelcome distraction to the task in hand and so we do not give it the priority it deserves. Curiosity is the essential element that powers our development from infants to children to adults. It is this driving force that enables us to discover the world in which we live.

When you allow yourself to satisfy your curiosity by exploring and seeking information, you reward your curiosity. That reward is highly motivating and, as a consequence, your curiosity will increase and you will discover more. Not only will this expand your knowledge in a beneficially chaotic and random way, which stimulates the brain to sort and match information, but understanding new ideas and concepts will greatly enhance your cognitive abilities. Next time you are ever so slightly curious about anything, make time to take a journey of discovery. Not only will you find the experience extremely satisfying and pleasurable, but you will also give your brain a powerful boost.

Lifestyle and the brain

Alcohol

When consumed sensibly and in moderation, alcohol makes a major and pleasurable contribution to our lives, but it is not without risk and, in the case of sustained heavy drinking, alcohol can have a significant detrimental effect on the brain. Alcohol will cause brain tissue to contract and permanently destroys brain cells.

Thiamine deficiency is a condition associated with heavy drinkers. Thiamine, also known as vitamin B1, is an essential nutrient required by all tissue and the most common source is meat and whole grains. The cerebellum lies underneath the brain and is responsible for coordinating movement as well as some forms of learning, and is the part of the brain that is most affected by thiamine deficiency. Thiamine deficiency will also affect memory and cognitive abilities in general.

Remember, it is good to drink but only in moderation.

Sleep

I have an unfortunate habit of leaving it until it is too late before I work out how much sleep I need. It is normally when the alarm clock goes off that I realise I should have gone to bed at least a day earlier. This is not because I treat sleep more casually than it deserves, but because I have the circadian rhythms of an 'owl' and my body clock is about an hour behind that of my wife, who is a 'lark'. Waking up to my wife's alarm clock is the price I pay for sleeping with the woman I love!

Good sleep is essential to the wellbeing of mind and body, and plays a vital part in enabling our brain to be the lean, mean, reasoning machine that powers our life forward. The reasons for sleep are many and include regulating autonomic nervous activity such as heart rate, enabling the brain to perform memory consolidation, and also regulating nerve cell activity to help prevent the nervous system from being overloaded.

The real benefits of sleep are paradoxically made more noticeable by the lack of it, and this cannot be illustrated more effectively than by a study undertaken in 2000 by researchers in Australia and New Zealand to ascertain the effect of sleep deprivation on driving[10]. The study concluded that lack of sleep had the same hazardous effect as driving while drunk, and the hazard increased according to the amount of sleep deprivation. After sixteen hours awake, driving performance began to deteriorate, and after twenty-one hours without sleep, driving performance was as bad as driving while over the blood alcohol limit. Sleep also has a profound effect on our ability to assimilate complex information, and for innovative thinking and decision-making[11].

Our sleep patterns are governed by our biological clocks. Our circadian timing system is a function of our genes and we all have a central 'biological' clock located in our brain. A key factor for regulating this clock is light, which synchronises our biological clock to the day-night cycle, which explains why it is harder to fall asleep in a well-lit room, even when it is late at night. However, if you have experienced even a moderate amount of sleep deprivation, it is hard to stay awake, even in bright sunlight. This desire to sleep is partially due to a neuromodulator called adenosine. Stimulants such as caffeine keep you awake by blocking the receptors to adenosine[12].

The best time to sleep is at night. Nighttime sleep results in lower body temperatures and higher concentrations of the sleep hormone melatonin. Melatonin, sometimes called the 'hormone of darkness', positively affects mood, therefore it is used increasingly in the treatment of a type of depression called Seasonal Affective Disorder (SAD).

The benefits of melatonin are numerous and include:

- Melatonin reduces cholesterol levels.
- It is a powerful antioxidant.
- It is linked with metabolism, and plays a part in weight control.
- Melatonin receptors are important in the mechanisms of memory and learning.
- Low levels of melatonin may be linked with Alzheimer's disease and some forms of cancer.

Nighttime sleep is also different in quality to daytime sleep. Nighttime sleep has more 'REM' sleep which is the type of sleep in which we experience most of our dreams. Another kind of sleep experienced more abundantly at nighttime is a deep sleep called 'sleep spindles'; it is during this type of sleep that memory consolidation occurs.

As we age, we tend to spend less time asleep, and to a large extent this is due to us requiring less sleep as we get older. In a study on sleep requirement, it was observed that when older volunteers were forced to stay in bed, they tended to stay asleep for an average of seven-and-a-half hours, and a study of those who lived longest reported that they slept between six and seven-and-a-half hours per night[13]. All this would indicate that a minimum of six hours' sleep is required for a long, healthy and mentally active life.

There is a gender difference in sleep patterns, with women enjoying a longer period of deep sleep, as well as sleeping longer – they also live longer! Recent studies suggest the female circadian clock is also about six minutes shorter than that of males, which may explain why they tend to go to bed and wake up earlier than men, and are often regarded more as 'early birds' in comparison[14]. This is fortunate for those women who believe they are from Venus because the planet, also known as the 'morning star', is at its brightest just before sunrise. Mars on the other hand is only visible to men at night.

Our circadian rhythms have a big influence on how we perform mentally and physically, and if we understand them we will get the most out of our hours, whether we are awake or asleep. An average person might experience the following typical circadian rhythm[15]:

02.00	Deepest sleep
04.30	Lowest body temperature
06.45	Increase in blood temperature
07.30	Cessation of melatonin secretion
08.30	Bowel movement likely
09.00	Maximum testosterone production for males
13.00	Least sensitivity to pain
14.30	Optimum coordination
15.30	Fastest reaction time
17.00	Greatest muscular strength and cardiovascular activity
18.30	Highest blood pressure
19.00	Maximum body temperature
21.00	Melatonin secretion commences
22.30	Bowel movements suppressed

Our circadian rhythms are controlled by a tiny pine cone-shaped patch of tissue, just above the optic nerve, called the suprachiasmatic nucleus (SCN). This body clock, the size of a grain of rice, is to a certain degree regulated and influenced by light, especially light that tends towards the blue and ultraviolet end of the visible spectrum.

If we want to get the most out of our magical body clock, we should reinforce it by the way we use light. Consequently, a small fifteen-minute dose of sunlight on the naked eyes as early in the morning as possible not only helps to boost serotonin levels but also resets our body clock.

Equally the human body, complete with circadian rhythms, evolved before artificial lighting was invented and at nighttime modern bright lights, especially the full spectrum variety used to treat SAD, can conflict with our body clock. This is especially significant as the night progresses. At about 9pm in the evening, the body expects to produce melatonin in anticipation of nighttime sleep. Exposure to strong light, especially the fluorescent light emitted from modern energy-saving light bulbs, can have a tendency to disrupt that process.

If you are one of those happy people who regularly feel that the day is just beginning at 9pm, try changing your evening lighting to a source that emits a softer and more yellow light. There is a reason for yellow being mellow.

Feeding the brain

The relationship between diet and learning has been the subject of a lot of research in the last decade, and the pace and quantity is increasing. So far, the majority of research has focused on the role of essential fatty acids, especially alpha-linolenic acid and linoleic acid. The results are increasingly emphasising the importance of these fatty acids together with the non-essential fatty Acids DHA and DMAE. Non-essential fatty acids can be manufactured by our bodies, however dietary intake is recommended to ensure that the optimum quantities are available.

All of these fats, essential and non-essential alike, can be obtained from oily fish, so grandmother really was right; fish is food for the brain. Although oily fish is top of the list, other good sources are nuts and seeds, root vegetables, red and white meat and nearly all green vegetables. A more specific explanation of the power of food is given in *Essential 5: 'Eating for health'*.

The dos and don'ts of a healthy brain

Do:

- Always learn to do something that is new. Anything will do, providing you have never done it before.
- Find time to do things the long, slow and hard way. Don't look at the answers or use a calculator.
- Have variety in your leisure activities.
- Enjoy finding and solving puzzles.
- Have conversations with other people. If possible, talk about ideas rather than other people.
- Get enough sleep.

Don't:

- Try not to watch television for the sake of it. It will sedate the brain and destroy it as certainly as sugar will destroy your body. There is a value to watching television, but only if the mind is actively engaged with the content. A book is a more stimulating way of passing the time. Better still, learn to play the bagpipes tunefully and quietly. It is the greatest unfulfilled challenge that still exists. The world will thank you.

Essential 4:
The importance of the body

In order to achieve immortality, we need a body that is fit and capable.

I am pleased, if somewhat surprised, with how fit I have become. I am definitely a lot fitter than I thought I would be when, six years ago, I first started training in mixed martial arts. Now I can spar for three-minute rounds without suffering too much damage, with youngsters one-third of my age. I can perform a routine consisting of fifty squats, fifty push-ups and fifty crunches without emergency medical assistance. At sixty-two years of age, I have much the same range of movements that I had when I was twenty-two. However, there are some things that are not the same; the joints protest at times, and I have learnt to my cost that my eyes don't focus on incoming boxing gloves as quickly as my nose would like. On the other hand, there are compensations; I can stay calm under pressure and I have stamina and endurance that allows me to outlast many of my opponents.

My fitness may be a personal achievement that gives me a lot of satisfaction, but it is modest when compared with the achievements of others. Dancing is perhaps one of the most physically demanding activities, yet some of the greatest performers continued to dance long after most other athletes have ceased to be television commentators. Dame Margot Fonteyn, Prima Ballerina of the Royal Ballet, did not retire from the company until 1979, at sixty years of age. When, in 1988, she danced for the last time with Rudolf Nureyev; she was sixty-nine years old, Nureyev was fifty years old, and another principal performer, Carla Fracci, was aged fifty-two years.

There are other athletes who are exceptional for carrying on long after most others have retired. Oskar Swahn, the Swedish marksman, won two Olympic gold medals at the age of sixty, and continued competing, winning an Olympic silver medal when he was seventy. However the prize for keeping going, in his case rather quickly, belongs to Philip Rabinowitz, who entered the Guinness Book of World Records when, on 10th July 2004, he became the fastest centenarian to ever win the 100 metres sprint.

Age is not a barrier to becoming and staying fit.

Effort and exertion are unavoidable if you wish to become fit and to get your body into shape. It is true that you can get into a shape watching TV, in the same way as you can get into a shape in a burger bar, but it will be the shape of a large maris piper rather than a lean, keen, long-living machine – even if you wear the trainers and tracksuit! The good news is that you will get into a pretty reasonable condition, and the shape of at least a junior league superhero, by doing things you can enjoy.

The essential goal of any fitness regime is to help the body to become fit and healthy, so we need to achieve a good heart rate and circulation, together with a general efficiency of the body. Alongside this, the ability to be physically capable of a wide range of activities, and an increase in stamina and strength are important goals. I am not a great advocate of prolonged exercise that burns you out, unless you want to join the Special Forces or compete in the Olympic Games. Extreme and punishing exercise is not necessary for the levels of fitness you need to achieve, and extreme exercise can carry a high price. It is potentially damaging to constantly stress the body for prolonged periods, and it can precipitate excess production of cortisol, which will accelerate the ageing process.

The desired fitness program is one that brings life-extending good health and a physical capacity to live life to the full. A welcome by-product of a good fitness program is not just feeling your best but also looking wonderful. Just watching the ladies smile when they set their eyes on aerobics fan George Clooney should be sufficient evidence!

The benefits of exercise on health and mind

There is a vast amount of convincing statistical evidence of the benefits of exercise on physical and mental wellbeing. The NHS, the guardians of the nation's health, list on their website the following benefits of about thirty minutes of moderate intensity exercise per day:

- up to a twenty per cent lower risk of breast cancer
- a thirty per cent lower risk of early death
- a thirty per cent lower risk of falls (among older adults)
- up to a thirty per cent lower risk of depression
- up to a thirty per cent lower risk of dementia
- up to a thirty-five per cent lower risk of coronary heart disease and stroke
- up to a fifty per cent lower risk of type 2 diabetes
- up to a fifty per cent lower risk of colon cancer
- up to a sixty-eight per cent lower risk of hip fracture
- up to an eighty-three per cent lower risk of osteoarthritis

All of these benefits are available without having to take a single pill and, unlike medication, the only side effects of moderate exercise are good side effects.

In 1999, the Duke University Medical Centre in North Carolina found that treating major depression with aerobic exercise was just as effective as using medication. What surprised them, however, was that the group which was treated using aerobic exercise demonstrated significant improvements in the mental processes of memory as well as the executive functions such as planning, organising and multi-tasking.

The benefits of exercise to health are compelling. However exercise becomes essential when you take into consideration the added enjoyment of being physically and mentally capable of living your life to the full. Before we look at the activities we need to do, we need to look at what we want to achieve from our exercises and why.

Maintain and extend the range of movements

This is probably self-explanatory, but it means being able to do in ten years' time what you used to do ten years ago, without hearing the painful sounds of pulling muscles or tearing ligaments. The exercises needed to do this are stretching exercises, which can be incorporated into some fun activities. Stretching exercises are an important stimulus for the body's growth hormones, so expect to be healthier, stronger and more youthful. Stretching is essential if you want to move like a teenager, and although it won't make you look like one, it's great for stimulating good skin. Some stretching routines are explained in the paragraph on stretching that follows.

Improve and maintain cardiovascular and lung capacity

By and large, it is difficult to achieve this without breaking into a sweat, but there are choices and a wide range of activities, some of which you will find good fun. As an added advantage, these exercises will also improve brain function, increase stamina and do wonders for your sex life, which for most people is a great incentive and, for some lucky people, highly motivating.

Effortful exercise is also a great way of stimulating adrenalin and endorphins, so expect to feel really good even if you are a little out of breath. Because cardiovascular exercise improves circulation, you will notice that your skin will thicken and glow with health.

I have a thing about capability. As a rule, I would rather be as fit as someone ten years younger than someone ten years older, so when I get to train with somebody, I try to train with someone younger, and let youth be my performance benchmark. Meanwhile, the youngster no doubt relishes the opportunity to be mentored in the fine arts of cunning and treachery! When I monitor my heart rate, I like to do a little high intensity training and get my heart rate into the range of the age group fifteen years below mine for thirty seconds or so. I will do this maybe four or five times during a half-hour session. It works for me; I think the human body responds to the pressures it needs to meet.

There is a paragraph on the benefits of high intensity training later in this chapter. However, before you undertake this, make sure that you do not suffer from any heart problems, and if you have the slightest doubts whatsoever, go and see your doctor and seek their advice.

Mind-body coordination

The first time I realised how really useful mind-body coordination is was probably the last time I watched adults run in a three-legged race. It was held on a small lawn and consequently involved two right-angle turns. The race was only over about a hundred yards, but somehow lasted two minutes, with only one pair making the finish line. The carnage was reminiscent of the chariot scene from 'Ben Hur', although fortunately, in this case, no horses were hurt and most of the contestants survived.

We take mind-body coordination for granted every time we turn a corner without tripping over our feet, and it gives us the confidence to be physically active and adventurous. It is also good exercise for the mind. Most competitive team sports require good mind-body coordination as well as activities as diverse as juggling, dancing, surfing and skiing. A spin-off benefit of these activities is that it often involves interaction with other people, especially when you practice juggling with cricket balls next to your neighbour's conservatory.

Strength

Strength does what it says on the tin; we no longer have to carry a dead bison back to our cave for dinner, but we need strength for everyday tasks like turning our mattress or unscrewing the lid on a jar of coffee. Strength is all about capability; the stronger you are, the more things you are able to do.

Exercise for strength is good for stimulation of testosterone and growth hormones, and is also a great way to keep the bones strong. By and large, the only way to get and maintain muscle strength is to load effort on the muscles, but there are plenty of fun activities that do this, such as swimming and rowing. Bones really respond to taking loads and impact activities, so most activities that build muscle strength will build bone strength at the same time.

Simple and easy exercises

There are a lot of exercises that you can do on your own that require no more equipment than loose clothing and a pair of trainers. These exercises are quick and simple, and don't require any more planning than allocation of time. In this group are stretching, running, cycling and walking. At the other end of the scale are team sports, which normally require a fair degree of organisation and some specialist kit. Below is a list of simple and easy activities and what they achieve.

Deep Breaths

I punctuate my exercises with five deep breaths. I really mean deep breaths. I suck in a roomful of air and let it out slowly. Breathe in through the nose – the hairs in the nostrils make great fly filters – hold for a few seconds, and then breathe out slowly through the mouth. Help your chest expand as you breathe in by lifting your elbows up into wings and pinning them back behind your shoulders, and then lower them as you exhale. When done properly, this a very exhilarating exercise. I always start my day with some deep breaths and stretching, and it's a great way to rediscover life the wrong side of a hangover.

Stretching

This is something that you can do on your own, and something I do every day. It requires a little space and about twenty minutes. Some stretches are best done when the body is warm. This means that some people prefer to do them after a jog, I prefer to do them when I've got out of a nice warm bed!

To do a full range of stretches, you need a space at least as big as a square of your stretched out body length. Start with something easy and progress to bigger extensions as your body warms up. When you stretch, it is important to work with your body. Don't expect to be as flexible with your first extension as you are with your last. Don't force your body; if you can't quite reach where you would like to, just repeat the stretch, and you will find that your range will gradually extend. Here is a list of the stretches I do but you might want to add others.

Toe touching: I normally start my stretching routine with thirty touches. I spread my feet about two feet apart, and touch alternate toes. After six touches, I try to touch the ground in the middle, between my two feet. Do this slowly and use gravity to gently help you to pull your body down until you can eventually touch the ground with your palms. It is a great way to start stretching routines.

Shoulder twists: Stand with your legs apart and your hands on your hips. Now twist your shoulders round, and alternate between twisting to the left and to the right. Twist as far as possible from the waist while keeping your hips immobile. If you are feeling ambitious, try doing this while doing your squats (see below). Some people prefer to place their hands behind their head rather than on their hips. Use whichever method is most comfortable for you.

Kicking: This is best done facing a mirror so that you can see how well you are kicking; however, don't stand too close unless you enjoy the sound of breaking glass. Stretch your right hand out in front of you, and kick out at your hand with your left foot. Each time you kick, raise your hand slightly higher so that eventually you, as an experienced immortal, will be kicking above head height. After fifteen kicks, change over so that you are kicking at your left hand with your right foot. This stretching exercise should leave you slightly breathless. If you haven't done this exercise before, you might find that you become a little sore and stiff. Don't despair! The stiffness will eventually disappear as you repeat the exercise over the next few days.

Arm flings: Stand with your legs slightly apart and fling your arms behind your body, then bring them back to cross over your chest. Really fling and feel those arms stretch out. Do this twenty times. Afterwards, you should feel slightly breathless if you have been putting the right amount of energy into this exercise. This is a great exercise for loosening muscles and will effectively relax muscles after weight training.

Neck rotations: This should be done gently, and under no circumstances should you force your neck to rotate. Stand securely and look straight ahead. Raise your chin up and stretch it towards the ceiling, then lower it to touch your chest. Rotate your face as far as possible to your left. Once again, raise your chin up then lower onto your shoulder. Now rotate your face as far as possible towards your right, and once again raise your chin up then lower onto your shoulder. Return your face to look straight ahead, and repeat the routine ten times.

Ankle pulls: The purpose of this is to stretch out the muscles and ligaments in the upper thighs, so expect a little bit of pain. Lay face down either on the floor or your bed. Reach behind you with your right hand and grab your right ankle. Now pull the ankle towards your bottom while keeping your hip bone pressed hard into the floor or bed. Pull until it hurts and then hold for thirty seconds. Repeat this three times, then change over and perform this routine on your left ankle with your left hand. This is one of those exercises that is working if it's hurting, so no pain, no gain! This exercise is best done when you are at your warmest, so I recommend that you leave this until the end of your exercise routine.

There are whole ranges of stretching exercises in use. The ones above are the ones I include in my daily routines, and they work for me. You might want to go and find some others. By and large, if it is attached to your body and it moves then it will benefit by stretching. However, never force your body into any position that it is reluctant to adopt, and if you are in doubt about the suitability of any exercise, you must consult your doctor.

Squats

I do twenty squats fairly slowly. Having trained with probably about a hundred people, I have discovered there are at least a hundred ways of doing a squat. The way I do them is to stand with my feet about twelve inches apart and clasp my hands behind my head. I then bend my knees and lower myself slowly into a squat or crouching position while trying to keep my torso as upright as possible. The challenge is to get as low as possible without falling over. When you have reached the low position, start to stand up and continue until you are perfectly upright. If you are doing the exercise correctly, your muscles will begin to hurt towards the end of your routine. If you haven't done any squats before, expect your muscles to feel a bit sore for the first few days. This exercise is also good for core strength.

Lunges

Lunges are a superb exercise for building muscle in the thighs, and strong thigh muscles shouldn't be the preserve of ice skaters. Every time you get yourself up from the floor, you use your thigh muscles. While most adolescents can get off the floor without using their hands for support, many adults can't, and this is due to body weight increasing and the strength of thigh muscles decreasing with age. The secret with lunges is to gradually increase the number of lunges you do over a period of a few weeks. If you reach the level of doing twenty lunges on each knee as part of your daily routine, you have reached the optimum.

For the uninitiated, a lunge is a curtsy with attitude. To do a lunge, stand with one foot about two feet in front of the other. Place your hands on your hips and go down on one knee until your knee is about one inch from the ground. Do not touch the ground with your knee. Hold this position for a count of five, then slowly raise yourself back to your original position. Repeat the lunge until you have completed five, then change stance so that the position of the feet is reversed, and then do five lunges on the other knee. Start at five lunges on each knee, and build to about twenty lunges on each knee over a period of a few weeks. It is normal for muscles to feel very sore when you first start doing this exercise; however the pain is well worth the gain!

Jogging

Jogging is a 'Marmite' activity; some people like it, others do not. I don't, although I am partial to Marmite. There are too many hills near me, which makes for hot hard work in summer and muddy misery in winter. I can't get my head around running in urban areas. By and large, the only people who look good jogging on the pavements don't need to jog, and those who need to jog should be hidden from sight. However, it's your choice and it gives a good cardiovascular workout. If you are scrambling down muddy mountains it is also good for mind-body coordination. Get a pair of good shock-absorbing trainers if you insist on doing this, as it can be quite punishing on the knees. Shock-absorbing trainers have specially designed soles and heels that absorb impact rather than transmit it to the ankle, knee and hip joints, and are widely available from most sports stores. It is not necessary to purchase the most expensive pair, as trials frequently show that the cheapest perform almost as well as the most expensive when running. If you are lucky enough to live in the countryside and like running off the beaten track, make sure you have a contingency plan to cope with injury. As a minimum, always take a mobile phone, kept dry in a sandwich bag, and wear high visibility clothing. If you like bouncing up and down on your knees and ankles but don't have a reliable sense of direction, you can always try skipping.

Skipping

This is another activity that you will either love or detest. It is, however, a great way to get a good cardiovascular workout. It does require a rope, and I recommend any skipping novice to enlist the help of a knowledgeable shop assistant when buying your first skipping rope. Size and weight make a huge difference to how well you will skip and consequently continue without either tripping over or slapping the back of your head with the rope. The latter can be hugely entertaining to anyone watching you, but after a while the head does feel a bit sore, which probably explains why bald men are either exhibition standard or don't skip at all. There are a huge variety of styles of skipping and they all yield approximately the same benefits. You will get a good workout from skipping three three-minute rounds with a minute's rest in-between. It is an effective way to strengthen the lower legs and ankles.

Walking

Walking can be a less miserable experience than jogging, as you can dress sensibly for bad weather. However, walking has to be done at a pace that gets the heart rate up if you aspire to a cardiovascular workout, so it's not ideal if you want to walk a dog with tiny legs at the same time. If you are not slightly breathless at the end of your walk, you have underdone the energy. The NHS website recommends two-and-a-half hours of moderately intense exercise per week for maximum benefit. Walking can be included in this exercise regime, but it has to be at sufficient pace so that, when you have finished, you feel slightly breathless and warmer, and your heart rate is a little higher.

Cycling

This is great cardiovascular exercise that is easier on the knees than jogging. It's also an effective method of building the strength of the lower body and, because it requires balance, it develops mind-body coordination. I have a bike, but I have to confess I don't use it much. The potholes and the manic traffic where I live sadly mean it's not the exercise of choice for those who want to achieve immortality. It is, however, an ideal form of exercise for those surrounded by good, safe roads or for those lucky to have access to a cycling machine. Always wear high-visibility clothes and a well-fitted helmet when cycling outdoors; however, I suggest slightly more discreet clothing for the spin class at your local gym.

Swimming

This is an enjoyable, and usually safe, method of cardiovascular exercise that is good for all-round strength. I would thoroughly recommend it to all those who like being in water, but as it requires a decent-sized swimming pool, it isn't always convenient. I used to swim a lot, and found it a fantastic way to become and stay trim. I would swim using both breast stroke and crawl techniques, and found both styles equally effective in building strength and muscle. When you swim, have either a time target or a distance target. Distance targets are great for beginners. When I started swimming, I would swim two thousand metres and constantly try to better my time. After a few months, my times came down sufficiently that I changed to a time target and consequently would try to swim the greatest distance in half an hour. Swimming requires very little equipment; I would however recommend using goggles as the chlorine in public baths can irritate the eyes, and a costume, as nudity in public baths can irritate the other users.

Exercise machines

These are great for cardiovascular workouts and for strength. It's obviously not the done thing for the purists, but I have a cycling machine that quickly converts into a rowing machine. It is easy on the joints and can be kept in the spare room, where I'm not in peril from manic drivers who haven't yet woken up from the night before. I'm also unaffected by the weather and can listen to the radio while swearing and sweating. Most exercise machines sold today have little computers that keep you informed about your session, including information about your heart rate. I can have a very good workout in thirty minutes that is good for strength, lung function and the heart. It can be a bit boring, but the radio helps and I'm warm and safe. If you don't want to buy your own machine or you prefer a bit of company, then nearly every gym has a large selection of exercise machines. Exercise machines are ideal for high intensity training as their heart rate monitors give you uniformly constant and accurate data to assess the intensity of your efforts.

High Intensity Training

The principle of High Intensity Training (HIT) is that a few short bursts of extremely intense effort can deliver most of the benefits obtained from longer periods of moderate intensity training[16]. This method, demonstrated by Dr Michael Mosley on the BBC's 'Horizon' programme in February 2012, involves getting on an exercise bike and pedalling gently for a couple of minutes and then going flat out for twenty seconds. This is followed by another couple of minutes of gentle pedalling to stay warm while getting your breath back, and then another twenty-second burst of flat out effort. This is then repeated for a third and final time.

This daily routine was followed for four weeks for the *'Horizon'* programme, at the end of which Dr Mosley was tested for insulin dependency. This was shown to have improved by a remarkable twenty-four per cent! The total time spent on exercise during this four-week period was thirty-six minutes of gentle pedalling and twelve minutes of intense flat out effort.

The effectiveness of this technique depends on the intensity of the effort. When you go flat out, you will use not just the leg muscles, but also the upper body and arm muscles. In other words you will activate eighty per cent of the body's muscles, compared to the twenty to forty per cent that will be used while jogging or walking.

I incorporate HIT into my training regime, but only do about three or four sessions per week. I use the heart rate monitor on the bike to measure my effort, and set my target heart rate for flat out effort at the maximum heart rate for a person ten years younger. In my case, my maximum heart rate should be about 160 pulses, and the heart rate of someone ten years younger is 170 pulses. I know when I have reached my target effort when the indicator on my exercise cycle exceeds 170 pulses, and I then maintain that effort for about twenty seconds.

Maximum heart rates will vary, but the average expected maximum heart rates for people of different ages are as follows:

- 35 years old: 187 pulses
- 40 years old: 182 pulses
- 45 years old: 177 pulses
- 50 years old: 172 pulses
- 55 years old: 167 pulses
- 60 years old: 162 pulses
- 65 years old: 157 pulses

I should stress that it is important to check with your doctor before commencing HIT.

Pilates

This is a great way to both stretch and build core strength. Don't expect to work up a sweat, but it is an effective way to keep your body doing things your mind would rather it didn't. I have never tried it, but my wife swears by it and gives me a detailed account of all the exercises she does each time she goes. A lot of the exercises sound like many of things I do at the martial arts gym, but done a little more genteelly and without the shouting and grunting. I am in no way suggesting that they hit people at pilates classes; if you want to do that, you need to join a martial arts gym or take up morris dancing.

Weights

Free weights are an effective way of building strength through performing repetitions under load. Exercises are specific to the muscles you want to work on and, as you have many muscles, there are a multitude of exercise routines. Because of this, I recommend that anyone who wants to use free weights uses a personal trainer to prescribe a routine of exercises according to their needs. Once the routines have been established, they are ideal for performing at home and, as weights are relatively inexpensive, they are an easy and affordable way to build considerable strength. Bench weights are not suitable for the inexperienced user to use at home and I would strongly recommend that anyone wanting to use them starts at a gym under the supervision of an experienced trainer. They are, however, the quickest way to build very powerful muscle, which is good for strength, endurance and looking good on the beach. If you want to build bulky muscle, you will benefit from nutritional supplements, and once again this is something best done under the supervision of an experienced trainer. Always stretch your muscles out after a weights session while the muscles are still warm.

Dancing

I've never been to dancing classes, but I can see the day coming when I will. Dancing can be incredibly energetic, so it will provide an excellent cardiovascular workout and the ultimate exercises for mind-body coordination. Needless to say, there will be a lot of stretching too. Vigorous dancing classes must rank as one of the best all-round workouts, so if you have a studio near you and are sufficiently uninhibited, I would recommend that you get involved. It must be the next best form of intensive workout after Mixed Martial Arts.

Martial Arts

Martial Arts covers a wide range of disciplines, from focused activities such as judo and karate to Mixed Martial Arts (MMA) where every discipline is used, so expect to kick, punch and wrestle on the ground. MMA involves full-contact sparring, which is highly energetic and, when properly supervised, is almost risk-free. Sparring in clubs is normally restricted to a light and continuous level, which should prevent the big guy from knocking lots of bits off you. However, expect to get hit, and expect a bit of pain when your enthusiastic opponent tires of trying to knock you to bits and decides to pull you to bits instead. It works very well for me as I have an aversion to being hit, so for three minutes I move with the speed of a frightened teenager and contort my body as I stretch, duck and weave. During a three-minute round I perform virtually every movement the body is theoretically capable of, plus a few more. The kick from endorphins and adrenalin is formidable. Wrestling is great for strength and stamina, and trying to land a kick while staying balanced and blocking your opponent's blows is the ultimate in mind-body coordination. For me, it ticks all the boxes and I would highly recommend it. An added bonus of MMA is that most syllabuses include self-defence, which is fun and an effective confidence booster. The cost isn't huge; there is the gym fee of about £50 per month, and my outlay on the kit is about £50 per year.

Solo sports activities

Solo sports include diverse activities such as surfing, skiing and horse riding. Most of these activities will involve a good amount of mind-body coordination, which will be enhanced considerably by counteracting the random challenges of nature. The amount of cardiovascular benefits will vary according to the sport, as will the amount of strength-building exercises. Costs will depend on the sport, but can be considerable.

Competitive sports

Competitive sports are a great way of enhancing mind-body coordination while having a cardiovascular workout. Team sports tend to provide opportunities for rest while other members of the team take the strain, and are also valuable opportunity to practice your social skills.

Competitive sports for the individual competitor tend to require higher levels of strength, stretching, cardiovascular exercise and mind-body coordination, some to almost lethal levels. I stopped playing squash several decades ago as a means of self-preservation. Some of my opponents were competitive well beyond their levels of competence or levels of fitness, which resulted in several matches ending quite spectacularly, and often accompanied by a modicum of anguish and pain. However, the advantage of any competitive activity is that you are motivated to extend your body, uninhibited by the limits of your mind, which produces great high levels of stretching, cardiovascular exercise and mind-body coordination.

Cramps

Some of us will live a life free of cramps, some of us don't. I'm one of those unfortunates who can be plagued by cramps, and the fear of them is always lurking at the back of my mind when training. Cramps are no more than a contraction or shortening of the muscles and are a consequence of muscle fatigue or deficiencies in sodium and potassium, but they are however extremely painful. I have tried many remedies for cramps and they all have a certain measure of success. By far the most effective is raising the limb above my heart, which normally involves me lying on the floor, and then massaging and stretching the muscle. If I can, I will make myself a lukewarm drink of sugar and water and drink as much as I can. I also find that taking a ZMA tablet every night reduces the incidence of cramps. ZMA was originally designed as a sports nutrition, and the tablets contain Zinc, Magnesium and Vitamin B6. There are a variety of manufacturers of ZMA and it available from most health food shops and sports stores, however before taking any supplements you should consult your doctor or a nutritionist.

The secret of exercise is to enjoy what you do, so choose carefully and you will be both happy and healthy.

The dos and don'ts of staying fit

Do:

- Stretch. Seize every opportunity to twist, bend and stretch.
- Do thirty minutes of intensive exercise per day. You must increase your heart rate and be at least a little breathless. The more you do, the fitter you will become.
- Improve your strength. Use weights, do push-ups, squats and lunges.
- Walk and carry rather than drive.

Don't:

- Do nothing!

Essential 5:
Eating for health

A good diet is essential for immortality. A good diet will give you health, energy and vitality.

Our relationship with food is unavoidable. If we do not consume it, we do not live. This does not mean that some people will attempt to live otherwise but, to date, no-one has succeeded and survived. Breatherists, as followers of breatherism are known, believe that life can be sustained by air and life-force alone and that no food is necessary. There are very few surviving breatherists, but of this few the most famous is Ellen Greve, or 'Jasmuheen' to her followers. In 1999, Jasmuheen, author of *'Pranic Nourishment – Living on Light'*, offered to let Australian TV monitor her for a week to demonstrate her methods. This offer followed an incident when journalists accidentally discovered that her house was exceptionally well stocked with food, which she explained was for the benefit of her husband. After four days of living on air and light, her pulse had doubled, she was over ten per cent dehydrated and had lost fourteen pounds in weight. The test was promptly stopped. This indicates that, even for breatherists, eating and drinking should be added to the list of things in life that are essential.

While Jasmuheen was demonstrating to an Australian audience the wonders of Pranic Nourishment, I was seeking an explanation for the mystery of my shrinking clothes. There was a short period of self-denial before I accepted the unwelcome truth that I would have to eat and drink less. This was followed by a period when I randomly started to cut down on consumption of anything that I thought might make me fat. For the shortest of moments, I contemplated following in Jasmuheen's footsteps, but was deterred by press reports that her dwindling band of followers was almost completely short of living members. Instead, I did what most of my friends were doing and tried to cut down on fats and sugars, and I was rewarded with an initial loss of a few pounds. Unfortunately, while losing weight, my skin tone became duller and I noticed that my energy disappeared. To make matters worse, my weight loss always seemed temporary and, despite the constant angst of attempting abstinence, I was never able to slide into my trousers without a deep intake of breath.

The next six months were devoted to experimenting with every diet I could find. With some diets I lost a little weight and with other diets I lost a little energy, with most of them I lost a little sanity. I found none of the diets sustainable and none of them made me glow with health.

With each new diet, however, I became increasingly curious and critical. I started to appreciate the importance of nutrition and I set out to understand all I could about what we eat, and what we need to eat, and why we need to eat it. I also started to experiment with vitamins and minerals and it wasn't long before my lethargy was being replaced with energy, and I detected a rather healthy vibrancy about my skin. What convinced me that I was going in the right direction was that my friends started to comment on how well I looked and started asking me about what I was doing. When my long suffering wife also confessed to noticing a change for the better about me and asked me what supplements she should be taking, my enthusiasm received a boost and I extended my experimentation to include the high-fat, low-carbohydrate diets that were just becoming available.

Within about six months, I had settled on a hybrid diet that was part Atkins and part Sears – The Zone. These diets restrict carbohydrates but their most controversial aspect is that they don't depend on restricting fat intake and, in fact, talked about the benefits of consuming specific fats. Dr Atkins provides a convincing argument that the best way to reduce cholesterol and lose weight is to go on a low carbohydrate diet. The benefits include an increase in High Density Lipoprotein, which is a good type of cholesterol that protects the heart, and a reduction in Low Density Lipoprotein. Low Density Lipoprotein, the villain of the cholesterol world, increases the risk of heart disease. The diet was also very effective in reducing triglycerides which is the form in which our body stores fat.

But Dr. Atkins wasn't the first person to make the association between heart disease and diet. In 1927, Thomas Cleave joined the Royal Navy as a Surgeon Lieutenant and began a career that saw him reach the rank of Surgeon Captain during the Second World War. In the course of his service, he travelled the world, especially to the countries that at that time made up the dominions, colonies and protectorates of the British Empire. Because of his travels, he was able to gain first-hand knowledge and understanding of the various health problems around the world and he found that certain diseases, especially heart diseases, were significantly more apparent in those colonies that were most westernised. But the western-type diseases weren't just restricted to heart problems, but also to the majority of conditions that are related to blood sugar levels, including diabetes. Dr. Sears picked up on Cleave's observations, and his Zone diet pays special attention to the way in which our hormones are affected by the things that we eat. Our hormones have a tremendous effect on our performance; they affect our mood, our energy levels, our libido and our general health. Using diet to control our hormones and keep them at their desired levels has a tremendous impact on us performing at our best.

Doctors Atkins and Sears were not the last people to promote high-fat low-carbohydrate diets. In 2008, the Swedish Public Health Authority endorsed a high-fat diet for citizens, in response to having one of the fastest-growing rates of obesity in Europe. Four years later, in 2012, it is estimated that one in four Swedes follow a high-fat low-carbohydrate diet, and the rate of increase in obesity has slowed to such a level that the Swedes are set to replace the Swiss as the slimmest people in Europe. Following the diet on such a scale was not without incident. During the run up to Christmas in 2011, the high demand for butter precipitated a butter shortage throughout Scandinavia. This shortage was especially acute in neighbouring Norway, where the price of butter momentarily reached over £200 per kilo, and three Swedes were arrested for smuggling butter across the border.

Diet has a tremendous effect on our appearance. Apart from the obvious issues of being the desired weight, healthy bodies tend to look healthy and that is because their skin is vibrant. High blood sugar levels may lead to glycation, a process where sugar reacts with proteins like collagen in the skin. When this occurs, the collagen becomes tough and inflexible making it more susceptible to the signs of ageing. As well as glycation, spikes in blood-sugar levels can cause fluctuations in adrenalin, and consequently testosterone levels, and this can aggravate acne and precipitate acne breakouts. There are only benefits in controlling your blood sugar levels to keep them low and stable. The skin also benefits from a diet rich in vitamins, minerals and antioxidants. The latter are essential in mitigating the ageing effects of ultraviolet radiation and other forms of environmental stress.

The problem I encountered with all of these diets is that they were high maintenance with regard to the amount of effort required to maintain them. This is fine during the early stages when there is a tendency to be enthusiastic to the point of obsession. However, we all have to live in a world where we socialise with friends, eat at restaurants and shop at supermarkets. This led me to find a set of dietary principles by which I could eat for optimum health and still participate as a relaxed, happy and social member of the human race.

The next step in the evolution of my diet came when I was introduced to the Palaeolithic diets. These diets are based on the foods available to our hunter-gatherer forbearers and have one simple principle; humans should avoid eating food that cannot be safely eaten in its natural, raw and unprocessed state. This principle is applied whether or not – and if, or how – the food is cooked before consumption, and it is used as the method to select the most suitable nutrition. I was surprised by how well I felt when eating foods selected according to this principal and, as this diet was based on choice of food rather than quantities of food, it was very easy to sustain.

All of these diets were, however, substantially dependant on identifying what we shouldn't be eating. What was needed was a diet that utilised the latest information about nutrition as the basis to select food purposely to optimise our health and, at the same time, enjoy all the available advances in agriculture. My experiments with vitamins and minerals had given me a very clear understanding of how nutrition affected our wellbeing, and so I set about adapting the low-carbohydrate and Palaeolithic diets to create a 'super diet' that was easy to follow but at the same time would provide the energy, health and vitality needed for immortality. I call it the *'Immortality Diet'*, because it provides the zing and zest for immortality.

The prime benefit of the Immortality Diet is that you will look and feel wonderful. The second benefit is that it is so simple it easily becomes a way of life, and consequently very sustainable. The third benefit is that there are very few absolute rules, just Very Good Foods, Good Foods, Foods and Bad Foods.

Whether a food is Good or Bad is determined by applying a simple test. This test is no more complex than ascertaining whether the outcome of eating a given food – apart from providing energy – is good or bad. Very Good Foods are those that you aspire to eat, and Very Bad Foods are those that you should eat only very occasionally, and examples are given later in this chapter. The Immortality Diet naturally steers you away from highly refined and processed foods that are normally nutritionally deficient or very high in simple carbohydrates, such as sugars. The diet also promotes fresh, seasonal and local produce. This introduces a variety of foodstuffs for you to eat that are at their nutritional best and, at the same time, reduces the risk of becoming sensitive or allergic to certain foods because of prolonged consumption. The Immortality Diet is fun and should be enjoyed.

There is a lot of jargon used when health professionals talk about nutrition, so it is perhaps worthwhile defining some of the more common terms before we discuss the diet in a little more detail.

Protein and amino acids

Protein is our only source of many essential amino acids. Amino acids are critical for life, and have a variety of roles in metabolism. Some amino acids are called 'essential' because the body cannot synthesise them and they can only be obtained from our diet. Not all amino acids produced by the body are beneficial in large quantities. Homocysteine is one such amino acid and high levels of these molecules are increasingly associated with cardiovascular disease and thrombosis. Homocysteine should not be confused with cysteine, which is a vital amino acid; it is suggested that one of the functions of cysteine is to reduce the toxic effects of alcohol and any resulting hangover.

The proteins in your cells can act as hormones, enzymes and antibodies to transport oxygen, vitamins and minerals throughout the body. Some proteins such as keratin and collagen are structural and are the building blocks of hair, skin and bones.

Animal protein is the most convenient source of all of our essential amino acids; however it is just about possible to obtain all of the essential amino acids from a vegetarian diet.

Vitamins and Antioxidants

Vitamins are organic compound nutrients that we require in tiny amounts that can only be obtained from our diets, as our bodies cannot synthesise them. Vitamins have many biochemical functions, such as hormones, antioxidants, cell signalling, growth regulators and precursors of enzymes. Vitamins are occasionally called micronutrients. In order for vitamins to be effective, they have to be consumed in a form that the body can use, or in other words they have to be 'bio-available'. Vitamins come in many forms, for instance there are five forms of vitamin D, but as a general rule dietary vitamins – vitamins in the food we consume – are bio-available.

Antioxidants are molecules that can prevent damaging oxidisation. The process of oxidisation can cause the production of free radicals, which can start cell-destroying chain reactions. The antioxidants in our diet remove and neutralise free radicals; they prevent these free radicals from rampant oxidation, which may damage other molecules, particularly DNA and other nucleic acids. Many antioxidants are also vitamins and vice versa. Vegetables are a good source of most vitamins and antioxidants. Fish and meat are also good sources and, in some cases, for instance certain B vitamins, meat is the only practical natural source. The most significant types of antioxidant are polyphenols all of which can be derived from plant sources.

There are over four thousand species of polyphenols, which include flavonoids and tannins, and although many have a beneficial function for the body, not all work as anti-oxidants. Research into the functions of polyphenols is in its infancy, but so far the results suggest that they may have many health benefits including anti-ageing, reduction in heart disease and inhibiting cancer. Tannins are used for their anti-bacterial and anti-viral properties. Polyphenols can be fun; the cocoa in chocolate is a source of polyphenols. However, nature is never as straightforward as we would like; phenols can be highly toxic and some plants contain members of the phenol family just to discourage animals from grazing upon them. This should not be of concern if you buy your vegetables from a greengrocer, especially one that depends on returning customers; look out for old customers that appear to know their way around the shop.

The role of vitamins in diets and their relationship to health remains very controversial. An inspection of the available data will show that every vitamin will have a range of medical conditions associated with its deficiency, with supporting evidence that ranges from epidemiology to specific clinical studies. The relationship between a deficiency of vitamin C and scurvy is perhaps one of the earliest epidemiological associations, and, more recently, the relationship between a deficiency in vitamin D and the bone disease rickets has received publicity. Equally, many vitamins can be shown to have a level of toxicity that will also be associated with medical problems. The medical profession is of two minds about the need and advisability of allowing the general public to have free choice in this matter, and will simultaneously discourage the use of supplements and yet prescribe vitamins for a variety of medical conditions.

For instance, folic acid, one of the B vitamins, is now almost universally recommended during pregnancy to reduce the risk of a multitude of birth defects. Despite this, the conservatism of the medical profession remains deeply rooted. In the last half of the previous century, Linus Pauling, the only person to win two unshared Nobel prizes, promoted 'orthomolecular medicine', the concept, which stated that optimum health could result from the right quantity of the right number of micronutrients in the body[17]. In 1973, he published *'Vitamin C and the Common Cold'* which contained the results of all of his research data. The book was a sensation, and convinced millions of Americans to take vitamin C. The medical community, however, were not so impressed and successfully attacked both Pauling's findings and his credibility. Fortunately today, some forty years later, his work has been re-evaluated and it is now largely accepted by the medical profession that originally rejected it.

Most of the negative issues concerning nutritional supplements will be avoided if single vitamins are not taken in isolation. Vitamins often work in conjunction with others and supplementing with a single vitamin may cause a deficiency in another. The safest way to take supplements is to take a multivitamin that removes the risk of inducing any such deficiencies. I would always recommend that you discuss your individual needs with a nutritionist before taking supplements. However, the best way by far of ensuring you have the desired levels of essential micronutrients is to have an optimised diet – the Immortality Diet.

The most significant vitamins are:

- **Vitamin A** comes in many forms of which retinol and beta carotene are the most significant. Vitamin A is an oil-soluble vitamin that is needed by the retina of the eye. It has a significant function for vision, gene transcription, bone growth, immune system and skin. It is also a powerful antioxidant. The retinol form is more commonly obtained from animal products and the beta-carotene is obtained from vegetables. The human body is not efficient at digesting beta-carotene and processing, for instance cooking, is needed to make it capable of being absorbed. Because this vitamin is fat-soluble, it will be stored by the body and it is possible to accumulate toxic quantities. However, you would have to try very hard to ingest toxic quantities of liver, but it would be worthwhile cutting back when you start looking like a carrot. The liver of the polar bear should be avoided, however hungry you feel, as it can have toxic quantities that may kill you before you look like a carrot. Hungry polar bears are best avoided altogether.

- **Vitamin B** comes in eight forms, although these forms are often found in the same foods. They are thiamine, riboflavin, niacin, pantothenic acid, pyridoxine, biotin, folic acid and cyanocobalamin. B vitamins are water-soluble and support the immune and nervous systems. These vitamins also support cell growth and division, and maintain healthy hair, skin and muscle tone. The body does not store B vitamins and toxicity is unusual from a normal diet. B vitamins are found in vegetables, seeds, nuts and other unprocessed whole foods, but are more concentrated in meat and fish. Vitamin B12 – cyanocobalamin – is normally only found in meat products, therefore vegans need to take supplements to ensure that they get an adequate supply of this vital micronutrient. Recent research suggests that the B vitamins may regulate levels of homocysteine, and help change this naturally occurring and harmful amino acid into helpful compounds. High levels of homocysteine in the body are associated with cognitive decline and cardiovascular disease. B vitamins are not normally associated with toxicity; however it is important that there is sufficient dietary intake of all eight forms to avoid the masking of deficiencies.

- **Vitamin C** is also known as L-ascorbic acid or L-ascorbate and is a powerful antioxidant. Vitamin C is necessary for the production of collagen, and plays an important role in wound healing and the prevention of bleeding from capillaries. A deficiency of Vitamin C can cause scurvy. This vitamin is very important for a good skin as it helps prevent or slow down damage from exposure to the sun and is needed for the immune system to function efficiently. Vitamin C is water-soluble and it is highly unlikely that sufficient of this vitamin could ever be consumed to be fatally toxic.

- **Vitamin D** is known as 'the sunshine vitamin' due to the ability of the skin to synthesis this vitamin when exposed to the shorter wavelengths of ultraviolet light known as UV-B. The reduced amount of sunshine in the northern hemisphere results in reduced amounts of vitamin D being created by the body, and the consequent deficit has to be remedied by dietary intake. It is unlikely that a person could consume and synthesise enough of this vitamin to reach a toxic level. More information on the benefits of this vitamin is given in the final chapter, *Essential 7: 'Enjoy the sun, nature's free tonic'*.

- **Vitamin E** refers to a group of fat-soluble compounds, the most common form of which are tocopherols, and are found abundantly in most cereal-derived oils, nuts and plant seeds. It is a powerful antioxidant and works best in this role in conjunction with vitamin C. This vitamin can act as an anticoagulant and high levels may increase the risk of bleeding, a condition known as hypervitaminosis E. To avoid this condition, it is recommended that the daily dose does not exceed 1,000mg. To put this quantity into context, it is a lot and would only be possible if, on a daily basis, you consumed in excess of either four kilograms of almonds or twenty kilograms of spinach.

- **Vitamin K** is a fat-soluble vitamin that is necessary for the coagulation of blood. The most significant dietary source of this vitamin is leafy green plants such as brassicas. It is unlikely that this vitamin can be toxic.

Minerals

These are the chemical elements essential for life, other than hydrogen, carbon, oxygen, sulphur and nitrogen. Most are normally only required in minute quantities and it is worth noting that of the sixteen minerals most frequently cited as being essential to life, too much can cause as many problems as too little. The six minerals we require most of are potassium, chloride, sodium, calcium, phosphorous and magnesium. Most foods are a source of minerals.

Essential fatty acids

The human body can produce all but two of the fatty acids it needs, and these are called essential fatty acids. Essential fatty acids (EFA) are polyunsaturated fatty acids that are used in the body to produce a range of hormone-like substances that regulate a wide range of vital functions; these include blood clotting, blood pressure and blood lipid levels, the immune response and the inflammatory response to injury infection.

A western diet is typically richer in omega-6 fatty acids than omega-3 fatty acids but, for optimum health, a diet should be richer in omega-3 fatty acids. The most commonly known and available omega-3 fatty acids are ALA, EPA and DHA. Oily fish and olive oil are good sources of EFA.

Glycemic Index (GI)

The Glycemic Index, often referred to as GI, is a measure of how much the level of blood sugar is raised by the consumption of a gram of carbohydrate contained in a particular food. The measure is relative to consuming a standard quantity of pure glucose, which has a GI of 100, and by comparison the carbohydrates in most other types of food – white bread can have a GI of 100 – will have a lower glycemic index. The glycemic index is used in the calculation of the glycemic load. A list of typical glycemic index scores for a range of foods is given in Appendix A.

Glycemic Load (GL)

The Glycemic Load (GL) is a number that indicates the expected increase in blood sugar levels that are a consequence of eating a certain food, and takes into account the amount of carbohydrate that is contained in the food and the speed at which its sugar is absorbed into the blood. For instance, a fruit such as a water melon has a high glycemic index because there is a high sugar content in the carbohydrate, but because a water melon contains a great deal of water – which has a GI of zero – and the carbohydrate is slowly absorbed, it has a low GL. Blood sugar levels are more likely to remain stable when eating foods with a low GL, which makes it an essential aid to controlling the effects of diabetes. GL is also a very useful tool when the prime purpose of dieting is to lose weight, in which case the GL of the foods consumed needs to be kept below 20. A list of typical glycemic loads for a range of foods is given in Appendix A.

The Immortality Diet: The perfect diet

- Simple to understand, easy and fun to follow.
- Very natural; it emphasises local, seasonal and unprocessed food.
- Good for health, weight control, skin and staying young.
- Requires no special food and you can eat as much as you want.
- This diet is ideal for 21st century life, and you don't need rise at 5am to go elk hunting and berry picking.

There are just six simple rules – it really is that easy!

Rule one: Eat local produce

This has many advantages. For the eco-warrior, it takes another lorry off our roads and reduces our carbon footprint. For the serious foodie, it has serious health-giving benefits.

Local food has a better chance of being really fresh. Fresh food has more of its intended vitamins and anti-oxidants active when you consume it.

Because local food is fresh, it is likely to have been picked when perfectly ripe. Perfectly ripe food is at its nutritional optimum. Once again, this means a better source of vitamins and oxidants. Of course, there is the added advantage that perfectly ripe food tastes the best.

Local food is seasonal. There are many advantages to food being seasonal, the obvious one is that if it is grown as nature intended, it is likely to be as nutritional as nature intended. But there are many other benefits. By eating seasonal food we will vary our diet, which will ensure that our diet includes the widest range of nutrients. Seasonal food also means that there are times of the year when we abstain from certain foods, and this will help to reduce the risk of becoming sensitive or allergic to certain foods.

Rule two: Eat variety

Variety enables you to benefit from the nutritional strengths of all of the foods available. Some foods will be rich in vitamin A, others might be rich in vitamin E and so on, but unless you include them all in your diet, you will never enjoy the benefits of an intensely nutritious diet. Go for a variety of deep, vibrant colours when choosing fruit and vegetables. Different colours usually indicate different anti-oxidants and as each antioxidant has its own particular benefit, the more types you enjoy the healthier and happier you will become.

Rule three: The raw test

If the food is poisonous in its raw state, man wasn't designed to eat it. Neither was woman. Some of these foods have now become accepted staples in our western diet, especially potatoes and legumes. Legumes are beans and other such podded fruit of the pea family, and include peanuts, soy and lentils. Such foods can be eaten as a treat but shouldn't be relied on as a staple of the diet.

The raw food test doesn't mean that all foods are best eaten raw. Some foods need cooking in order for humans to digest them, such as root vegetables. Carrots, for instance, are best eaten cooked if you want to obtain the vitamin A within them, and meat is more easily digested when cooked. There are also other important hygiene reasons for cooking food; it kills unwanted bacteria, a process that enables us to eat our food, sleep at night and wake up the next morning.

Rule four: Eat simple, eat unprocessed

Although there are occasions when processing helps to release nutrients within a food, it is usually best to eat food in its most natural state. Some intensive processing turns food into something best avoided. A good example of this are trans-fats, which are sometimes called hydrogenated vegetable oils, such as margarine. A typical trans-fat would be based on corn oil, which is in itself an oil obtained by an industrial process. The oil is heated to a very high temperature and combined with hydrogen using a metal catalyst and the result is a foodstuff unlike anything the body is meant to consume. Trans-fats are now associated with high cholesterol and heart disease. However good they might taste, you can always get nature to test them by putting a little outdoors on a plate next to a little butter and seeing where the flies chose to go. I have yet to see the flies chose the margarine, even the expensive 'good for you' brands.

Industrial processing is usually focussed on extracting a particular attribute from a food, regardless of the effect on the food as a source of nutrition. Refining is a good example. Refined white flower can render it almost nutritionally empty; it becomes a mere starchy bulking agent for making cheap white bread. It has been completely depleted of nutrients such as vitamins and minerals and has no fibre. When this white flour is combined with trans-fats to make pastry, it should be recognised for what it is: a high-energy comfort food that the body wasn't designed to eat, with a zero nutritional value.

Rule five: Beware sugar

Sugar gives food a sweet taste that most of us enjoy, however the enjoyment comes at a huge cost. Sugar is concentrated energy and its consumption is the surest way of piling on the pounds. Sugar will also have a bad effect on your health; every time you consume it, it will quickly boost your blood sugar levels, triggering the release of insulin and over time this will increase the risk of diabetes. High blood sugar levels will cause the creation of advanced glycation end products (AGEs). AGEs are likely to alter and damage proteins and are linked to many age related diseases. AGEs also deplete nitric oxide levels, which promotes vascular damage and an increased risk of heart disease.

Cavemen didn't have sugar – it rots the teeth!

Rule six: Eat Very Good Foods, do not eat Bad Foods

It is as simple as this. Below are lists of foods that will determine your diet.

a) Very Good Foods to be eaten as often as you can

Really Good Foods and Good Foods in the next category should make up seventy-five per cent of your diet.

- *Brassicas (cruciforms) in season, especially kale and tenderstem broccoli:* Brassicas include leafy green vegetables such as cabbage and cauliflower, and are rich in Vitamins A, C, E, K and folate. They are also a good source of fibre and provide resistance against cancers of the colon, rectum and thyroid. A wide range of phytochemicals –antioxidants – are found in brassicas, and they are increasingly associated with providing resistance to chronic diseases such as heart disease and cancer, and problems linked to ageing.

- *Oily fish, the smaller the better:* Although all fish is good, oily fish is very rich in essential fatty acids. Oily fish include sardines, herrings, mackerel salmon and trout. These fish contain high levels of omega-3 fatty acids and vitamins A and D. The benefit to general health of these nutrients is substantial, but they are especially associated with ocular and cardiovascular health and providing resistance to dementia. Anchovies, sardines and wild salmon are also a good source of DMAE, a substance found in small amounts in the brain that is associated with cognitive function. DMAE is also used in some upmarket skincare products to firm skin.

- *Tomatoes, including processed tomatoes, are really good:* Tomatoes are a rich source of lycopene and beta-carotene, a form of Vitamin A. Lycopene is an antioxidant found in the red pigment. Both Lycopene and beta-carotene are concentrated when tomatoes are cooked or processed, however this action will reduce the amount of Vitamin C available. Tomatoes are also a good source of Vitamins E, K and B6, folate, potassium, magnesium, phosphorus and copper. Tomatoes provide a certain degree of protection from ultraviolet radiation and cancers including colon, prostrate, breast, lung and pancreatic tumours.

- *Asparagus:* Asparagus contains high levels of folic acid and vitamin C, together with good levels of Vitamins A, B, E, K, phosphorous, potassium, copper, selenium calcium, magnesium, chromium and iodine. The root contains steroidal glycosides, which help reduce inflammation. About six spears of asparagus will provide about half the required daily intake of folic acid. Folic acid or folate is critical for pregnant women and may play a significant role in reducing levels of homocysteine.

  Asparagus is renowned for its distinctive 'bouquet' as it leaves the body. It is a smell that has attracted the attention of the famous throughout history; Shakespeare and Benjamin Franklin have written about it, although not in a complementary manner, and Marcel Proust more mischievously remarked that it *"...transforms my chamber-pot into a flask of perfume"*. The rogue ingredients are volatile organic compounds, which release aroma rich by-products, such as methanethiol or mercaptan, as it is digested. Do not be deterred or self-conscious; it is a fragrance that marks you out not only as a person who eats very healthily, but also as a person of impeccable dietary taste.

- *Berries:* A berry is any small edible fruit that doesn't have a stone, but may have seeds. This definition allows for a large variety of berries, each and every one having a unique combination of antioxidants, vitamins and minerals in both the skin and flesh. To obtain the greatest benefit from this wonderful source of nutrition, it is important to eat the widest variety according to seasonal availability. The skins of berries are particularly rich in compounds called polyphenols, flavonoids and tannins. These compounds are often excellent antioxidants. Berries are also an excellent source of carotenoids – vitamin A – and vitamin C. Examples of berries are grapes (red grapes contain the anti-ageing compound resveratrol), blackcurrants (very high levels of vitamin C and good levels of phosphorous, potassium and a lot more) and raspberries (vitamins C and B, together with very high levels of antioxidants). Although no studies have shown the effects against cancer of the antioxidants in berries, related studies on mice and other mammals suggest they have a strong preventative effect.

- *Unroasted, unsalted nuts and seeds:* Among the healthy nuts are almonds, hazelnuts, almonds, pecans, pistachio and pine nuts. Although they are called nuts, peanuts and cashews are legumes and are excluded from this list. Nuts can be a good source of omega-3 fatty acids, vitamin E, magnesium, manganese, zinc and phosphorous. Nuts make a great snack with no adverse effects on health and are a great source of essential minerals. To get the best benefit from nuts, eat a variety rather than restricting your selection to one or two types.

Seeds also make a great snack and, like nuts, can be very nutritious. Once again, eating a variety is important in order to get the full benefit. The nutrients found in seeds are many. They contain good quantities of vitamin E, minerals and omega-3 fatty acids. Hemp seeds contain good quantities of fibre as well as being a good source of protein. Sunflower seeds are a good source of phytosterols and folate, and also contain zinc and selenium. Phytosterols are a type of chemical found in plants that are similar to cholesterol; they are believed to control cholesterol levels and boost the immune system. Sesame seeds contain calcium, magnesium, zinc, fibre, iron, B1 and phosphorus. Pumpkin seeds are a good source of zinc and phytosterols. In fact, nearly every seed sold as a food is nutritionally wonderful and they can be consumed for both health and pleasure.

Seeds are surrounded by a protective casing that makes them difficult for the body to digest. Consequently, they should always be thoroughly chewed, otherwise they will pass straight through the body. Some seeds, such as linseed or flaxseed, are difficult to effectively chew because of their very small size, and you may find it advisable to blitz them in a coffee grinder before serving.

Nuts and seeds add flavour and texture to salads and stir fries.

- *Game (in season):* Wild game encompasses every type of mammal that hasn't been reared and that lives in the wild, such as pheasant, partridge, venison and wild duck. Game will always be seasonal, naturally-fed and free of antibiotics, steroids, hormones and preservatives. Wild game is very low in saturated fat and averages about one-seventh of the fat of farmed beef but, on the other hand, it is richer in essential fatty acids. Game can also be rich in vitamins C and E, and rich in antioxidants such as flavonoids and carotenoids. Wild game is rich in protein and is consequently an excellent source of essential amino acids.

b) Good Foods that should form the basics of your diet

Really Good Foods in the category above and the Good Foods in this category should make up seventy-five per cent of your diet.

- *Root vegetables, especially locally-grown beetroots and carrots:* Root vegetables – this excludes potatoes, which are tubers – have very little starch and are consequently a very good source of complex carbohydrates that will have a low GL score. A complex carbohydrate is a form of carbohydrate that is digested slowly. This enables root vegetables to be an excellent source of energy without having an adverse impact on blood sugar levels. Root vegetables include beetroots, parsnips, carrots and turnips, all of which are good sources of antioxidants, vitamin C, nitrate, magnesium, sodium and potassium. Of these roots, beetroot is exceptionally beneficial as it has very high levels of dietary nitrate, which supports the body in producing nitric oxide. Nitric oxide induces vasodilation and increased blood flow, and consequently enhances athletic stamina. Beetroot is also a good source of antioxidants and the compound betaine. Betaine works with other nutrients to reduce levels of homocysteine.

- *Freshly-picked ripe fruit – chose a variety of vibrant colours:* Fresh fruit is an excellent source of vitamin C and antioxidants. It is the ideal way to satisfy a sweet tooth without seriously elevating blood sugar levels. Fruit is best sourced from local growers, to ensure that it has been picked when ripe and that it is fresh. Water-based vitamins can degrade during storage, consequently a fresh and ripe piece of fruit will provide the most nutrition, and will also taste wonderful! Remember, however, that fruit has a high sugar content and that only a small amount of fruit, for instance one apple, should be consumed on a daily basis and, if you are trying to lose weight, it should be avoided completely; eat more salad and green leafy vegetables instead.

- *Fresh Salads – chose dark green and vibrant colours:* Salads can bring many of the nutritional benefits of brassicas. Like brassicas, salads are also a good source of minerals, vitamins and antioxidants. A salad item is any edible vegetable matter that grows above ground that can be safely eaten without cooking or processing. Salads, especially salad leaves, contain complex carbohydrates and have virtually no impact on blood sugar levels, regardless of the quantity eaten. They consequently are the ideal food for people who are eating to be trim and slim.

- *Fish:* Although white fish is not as rich in vitamin D and essential fatty acids as oily fish, it is still an excellent source of protein and nutrients. It is rich in B vitamins, iron, selenium and iodine. Shellfish is a good source of zinc. Zinc helps to maintain the functioning of cells and genes, and also supports wound healing and the immune system.

- *Avocados:* Avocados are a rich source of potassium, as well as providing high levels of B vitamins and vitamins K and E. Avocados also have a high fibre content. A high proportion of the fats in an avocado are monounsaturated, and the regular consumption of avocados has been shown to reduce harmful cholesterol. A study into the effects of an avocado-rich diet revealed that, after seven days, levels of triglyceride and harmful cholesterol – LDL, Low Density Cholesterol – fell by seventeen per cent within the test group, whereas levels of good cholesterol – HDL, High Density Cholesterol – increased by eleven per cent[18].

- *Onions, leeks and garlic:* These tasty members of the allium family are a good source of minerals, vitamins and anti-oxidants. They also add a delicious and satisfying taste to a wide range of food, and on that basis alone they earn their place in the good food category.

- *Red meat:* Red meat has received a lot of adverse press in the last two decades. It began with the BSE/VCJD, more commonly known as 'Mad Cow Disease', scare in the mid-1980s and continues today as a consequence of its association to certain cancers, especially bowel (colorectal) cancer. However, red meat is an excellent source of the B vitamins niacin, riboflavin, thiamine and B12, as well as all nine essential amino acids. Red meat is also a good source of iron, zinc and phosphorous; the kidney, heart and liver are among the best dietary source of Alpha Lipoic Acid, one of the most powerful antioxidants. Because of these superb nutritional properties, it should be included in the Immortality Diet. The risk of cattle suffering from BSE – bovine spongiform encephalopathy – has now almost disappeared as a result of improved farming practices. The risk to you, the consumer, is extremely small, however this small risk can be almost completely removed by eating naturally-reared and fed meat – this will include most British-reared lamb. The risk of bowel cancer can be reduced by high levels of vitamin D and an increased consumption of vegetables. The nutritional benefits of including a moderate amount – about 100 grams per day – of good red meat as a part of the Immortality Diet far outweigh the risks. Red meat is delicious.

- *Poultry:* Poultry includes chicken, turkey and farmed duck. I am very particular when I buy any form of poultry; I will only buy naturally-fed, free range poultry from a butcher who has visited the farm where the bird was raised. Free range poultry is less prone to disease and consequently will probably contain smaller quantities of antibiotics in its meat; it is also tastes better. Chickens are the most popular form of poultry and they provide an inexpensive but excellent source of protein. Chicken contains good quantities of vitamins, especially niacin and B6, and is an excellent source of selenium and phosphorous.

- *Eggs:* Eggs are the ultimate convenience super-food. Easy to store, quick to cook and delicious to eat, whole eggs have a high content of protein and the B vitamins. They also contain vitamins A, D and E, choline, phosphorous, iron and zinc, as well as all the essential amino acids. The nutritional value of eggs is very dependent on the quality of the diet of the laying hens, so buy the best eggs you can afford.

- *Dairy produce:* Dairy produce is an excellent food that has wrongly acquired a bad reputation as a consequence of the fashion for low-fat diets. Dairy products, especially full-fat products, are gradually being rehabilitated as health foods. The calcium in milk has a greater bioavailability – the ability to be absorbed – than calcium from certain vegetables such as spinach. It is also a good source of biotin, iodine, magnesium and the vitamins A, B, D and K. Low fat milk has a higher content of lactose – a sugar – than full fat milk and consequently it has a significantly greater effect on blood sugar levels. Skimmed milk also has significantly reduced levels of the fat-soluble vitamins A and D and consequently, for nutritional reasons, it should be avoided. According to a study in 2006, full-fat dairy products are likely to increase fertility in women, whereas low fat products reduce fertility[19]. Dairy fat also contains trans-palmitoleic acid and, in 2010, a 20-year study by the Harvard School of Public Health found that participants with the highest levels of trans-palmitoleic acid had a sixty per cent lower risk of developing diabetes compared to the other participants[20].

- *Most herbs and spices:* Herbs and spices are a great way to add flavour, and are increasingly being researched for their health benefits. However, the quantities you are likely to use in cooking are so low that any benefits and risks are negligible. I include them in this category purely because they make food fun.

- *Olive oil:* The oil of choice when butter isn't appropriate, you should use either the Extra Virgin or Virgin grades. These grades are produced by physical means without the use of any chemical treatment. Olive oil is good for both cooking and for use in salads, and is the only oil with which to make mayonnaise. It contains polyphenols and is rich in oleic acid.

c) Foods that can supplement your diet

These foods can constitute up to twenty-five per cent of your diet.

- *Legumes, in other words beans and other things in a pod:* Legumes are a good source of protein but, as there is a degree of toxicity with most uncooked legumes, they fail the Palaeolithic test. They are included in this category rather than the next as they are a good source of fibre and nutrition and on average have modest GL scores.

- *Whole wheat and other grains, including rolled porridge oats:* Whole grains refer to unprocessed grains. Processing them into flour increases their GL score to that of sugar, so beware. Rolled oats are a good source of protein and dietary fibre, together with iron and the B vitamin thiamine.

- *Wholemeal or wholemeal bread:* This is included because of its practicality; I have yet to see a sandwich made without bread, and sandwiches are a popular and convenient weekday lunch. Any bread, whether wholemeal or other, will have a high GL score. The effect on blood sugar can be reduced by spreading the bread with butter.

- *Wholemeal pasta:* Life would be dull if we were unable to indulge a passion for Italian food. However, any pasta has a high GL score, so always eat it with an oil-based sauce, and even then you should only eat it occasionally. Wholemeal pasta should not be confused with Giuditta Pasta, an Italian opera singer who died in 1865. Pasta was the favourite food of another opera singer, Luciano Pavarotti who, weighing just under one-sixth of a ton – allegedly – made as much of an impact on the scales as he did at La Scala.

- *Whole rice:* Whole rice is a good source of protein and dietary fibre. Whole rice, especially wild rice, is a good source of most B vitamins, iron, potassium, manganese, phosphorous and zinc, although it does have a high GL score.

- *Dark Chocolate:* Life is for living. Choose chocolate with more than sixty per cent cocoa solids and try not to eat more than seventy-five grams in a week. Good chocolate will contain antioxidants, just in case you need persuading.

d) Foods that are treats

You shouldn't eat more than one serving of any of the following foods in a week.

- *Potatoes:* Potatoes have a very high GL score and fail the Palaeolithic test; they share a toxin with other members of the deadly nightshade family. They do, however, provide useful nutrition.

- *White bread:* This is usually totally free of any nutritional purpose and will cause havoc with your blood sugar. I include white bread reluctantly, and only because the more social of us will visit friends and eat with them. If a friend ever invites you to dinner and gives you white bread, you should thank them with a copy of this book.

- *Pastry:* Unless you make your own with butter and wholemeal flour, this is yet another food with no nutritional purpose.

- *Refined white rice:* The refining process removes all nutrition, and white rice would be almost pointless were it not for Indian and Chinese food. Having said that, white rice is quite effective at removing moisture from salt shakers.

- *Peanuts and cashews:* These are legumes in disguise; but they are tasty, come in little packets and provide a good source of protein. I frequently succumb to temptation when I'm drinking beer. Unfortunately, I don't often drink beer.

e) Bad Foods, those that should have a health warning

These items are not food, and are just a means of perpetuating an addiction to sugar. Feel extraordinarily guilty if you do succumb to temptation! They will probably rot your teeth before they kill you, and are best suited to giving as presents to people you don't really like.

- *Sugar-based sweets including toffee and caramel.*
- *Most biscuits and cake.*
- *Fruit juices – they have high sugar levels and are very acidic.*
- *Fizzy drinks – any type of carbonated and sweetened drink.*
- *Margarine and other trans-fats.*

Drink

The average physically active male requires about two litres of fluid per day, a good proportion of which will come from the foods we eat. Females will require slightly less fluid. Tomato juice, tea and coffee have good levels of antioxidants. Beetroot juice is a great drink for boosting athletic performance due to its high nitrate content[21].

Caffeine has many benefits and should have a place in everyone's diet. The most recent study, publicised in July 2012, showed that increasing the amount of coffee consumed could lower the risk of skin cancer[22]. The researchers, led by Dr. Jiali Han, examined data from studies involving more than 112,000 women over twenty years and found that there was an inverse relationship between the incidence of basal cell carcinoma and the amount of coffee that was drunk. This research adds to a range of recent studies that have shown that coffee may protect against some illnesses, including type 2 diabetes, heart failure, Parkinson's disease, liver cancer and cirrhosis of the liver, and that it might improve exercise performance. If you're not a fan of coffee, drink tap water.

Alcohol is good. A little and often does have health benefits, whereas irregular and excessive consumption is harmful. Red wine is a good source of resveratrol and real ale has a few B vitamins. Spirits have very little effect on blood sugar levels. Moderation is the key and never, ever drink and drive.

For more on food, see *Appendix B* where you'll find a few great recipes.

Essential 6:
Looking the part

We like to look at others, and a lot of us like others to look at us. It is part of our evolutionary heritage to be aware of the way we and others appear. The subconscious mind of all animals is nurtured from birth to decide reflexively and instinctively whether a stranger could be a threat, a friend, a mate or food. Humans have, in addition, a capacity for self-reflection and consequently they also conjecture about how others see them. This creates two aspects of our appearance; the first is how others see us, and the second is how we see ourselves. Both aspects have a significant effect on the way we conduct our lives and our social interactions with others.

Some animals are known for their ability to change their appearance to give themselves an advantage in specific circumstances. Peacocks display their feathers to look healthy and powerful so that they might attract a mate. Cats arch their backs to appear big and strong so that they might deter aggressors. These are all instinctive reactions to suit immediate circumstances. Humans, on the other hand, will consciously adapt their appearance in anticipation of an almost infinite variety of possible future events. This trait has survived the rigours of evolution because it confers an advantage.

We can influence how we appear in many ways. When we deport ourselves with energy and a strong upright posture, others will perceive us as strong, energetic and in our prime. In most cases, our first impression of others will be based on deportment and physical posture. We further influence our appearance by means of superficial presentation, such as our clothing. We can choose to present a persona that may be fashionable, casual, conforming, iconoclastic, extrovert, modest or anything else that comes to mind by the clothes we wear, the way we cut our hair and the make-up we apply. Our appearance is also equally influenced by the quality of our skin, and good skin conveys health and vitality; again these are attributes associated with being in our prime of life.

Our skin is the human body's largest organ. It is vital to our life and serves many purposes. It protects us against the outside world by keeping out the environment, preventing excessive water loss and encasing our bones and other organs with a shock-absorbing layer. It helps our body to regulate temperature so successfully that we can exist and survive in a wide range of climates. It is a sensory organ that lets us feel when we touch, and consequently we can use our fingers and thumbs as precision instruments. The skin also enables us to detect temperature and pain so that we can keep ourselves safe. The skin produces vitamin D when it is exposed to sunlight. Our skin is wonderful.

Skincare is a new science. Before 1950, the only choice of skincare available to the majority of people was the choice between petroleum jelly and cold cream. Any defects that could not be remedied by these products were hidden beneath opaque layers of heavy make-up. Since then, the science of skincare has made huge advances. We now know how the sun and environmental factors can damage or age the skin and we also know how we can repair and prevent such damage. We have techniques that incorporate diet and topically-applied serums, and surgery is available should more dramatic remedies be required.

Cosmetic surgery is beyond the scope of this book. I can't teach you how to do it, although there is currently no legislation restricting your ability to perform surgery on yourself or others, should you find a volunteer. I do not recommend this. What you cannot do is prescribe anaesthetic or any other medication unless you are a doctor. For those of you who feel a need for surgery, then be very careful with your expectations. Cosmetic surgery is a good solution for dealing with specific and identifiable defects, for instance the shape of a nose, baggy eyelids and so on, but it has lower satisfaction rates for less tangible objectives such as anti-ageing facelifts. The average perceived reduction in age as a consequence of a face lift is about seven years, which is appreciably less than any expectation you may have gained from the 'Ten Years Younger' programmes shown on TV. When you choose a surgeon, make sure he is a Plastic Surgeon with recent, and successful, experience of performing the operation you require, and always obtain and take up references from clients who have had the same operation[23].

The rest of this chapter is about helping you to achieve a healthy and vibrant skin, giving you a few simple and easy techniques to protect and maintain it. Skin care is a way of life. It requires a good diet and a healthy lifestyle, as well as techniques for protection and cleaning. Good skin care will not only prevent further damage but will also encourage your body's own repair mechanisms to restore your skin to a more youthful and unblemished condition. Some damage, however, will require a little more than home care, and later in the chapter we discuss the types of specialist non-surgical treatments that are available, along with an indication of the results they can provide. To begin with, we are going to discuss what you can do yourself at home. The right home care is easy, inexpensive and very, very effective.

If you have been following the programme, especially the diet, you will have noticed a change in your appearance within the first two weeks. Being positive, fit and eating optimally will take years off your appearance. However, there is more that you can do to optimise your skin and let your youthful vibrancy radiate out for all to see. To do this, we need to embrace a skin care regime that will bring about anti-ageing skin rejuvenation.

Ageing is caused by internal (intrinsic or chronological) and external (extrinsic or environmental) factors. The results of ageing, regardless of cause, are the diminished production of collagen, which is the main supporting protein of the skin, and the breakdown of the elastin fibres, which give the skin its flexibility. Ageing is also accompanied by a decline in the activity of the sebaceous glands and this reduces the ability of the skin to retain moisture. A lack of moisture results in a reduction in the suppleness of the skin and also affects the ability of nutrients to reach the skin cells.

Good skin care will improve the quality of the skin by encouraging the production of elastin and collagen, and restoring the moisture content of the skin. This improvement in quality, coupled with the restoration of the skin to a pre environmentally-damaged state removes and reverses many of the visible effects of ageing. Anti-ageing skin rejuvenation is the process of returning the skin to a condition it enjoyed before it suffered damage or trauma during the passage of time. The characteristics of the type of damage are as follows:

- *Intrinsic (chronological) ageing:* This is sometimes referred to as chronological ageing and implies cellular degradation due to repeated replication of cells. This results in the skin getting thinner and less elastic. Intrinsic ageing is an inevitable, genetically-programmed process, the underlying mechanisms of which still remain largely unknown. The effects of intrinsic ageing on the skin are partially reversible. Intrinsic ageing is sometimes light-heartedly referred to as the effects of gravity and can be slowed down significantly by a good at-home skin care regime.

- *Extrinsic (environmental) ageing:* The degrading effects of the environment – including solar and other radiation – and lifestyle. Extrinsic ageing has many symptoms and can include thin, less elastic skin. Extrinsic ageing also includes a coarse rough texture, irregular pigmentation and broken capillaries – thread veins. Most of the effects of extrinsic ageing, especially photo ageing, can be substantially reversed by a good at-home skin care regime.

- *Illness and accidents:* This is typically manifested by scars, both pigmentary and by irregularities in the surface of the skin. The effects of scarring can be substantially reversed, but significant results will often require treatment at a skin clinic.

Good skin care will give you a great skin. However, good skin care is all about acquiring habits that you can sustain, because you have to be patient. To look great for a party tomorrow, for example, you'll need to have been looking after the skin for at least a month beforehand. Generally speaking, refining the surface of the skin is something that can be accomplished within two weeks, thicker collagen takes about two months and evening out superficial pigmentation can take up to six months. So the sooner you start, the sooner you will see the results.

We are going to commence with the basics of good skin care and then, later in the chapter, we will look at the conditions and blemishes that require slightly more specialised treatments, and the merits of the various treatments that are available in skin clinics.

There are three essentials to skin care; the first is managing the acid-alkaline – or pH – balance of your skin, the second is ensuring that it is adequately protected from ultraviolet radiation, and the third is gentle and regular exfoliation.

pH balance

To begin with, we will look at why the acid-alkaline balance (pH) of your skin is so important and why we have to manage it. The pH of your skin is the measurement of the acidity or alkalinity of the skin's surface. The measurement is on a scale of pH0 to pH14, where 0 is extremely acidic and 14 is extremely alkaline. Neutral is pH7, which is midway between the two points. When the pH is 7, the object of measurement is neither acid nor alkaline. Pure water has a pH of 7, and human blood is slightly alkaline with a pH of 7.4.

Measuring the pH of the skin's surface reveals a lot about the make-up of its outer layer, which is called the epidermis. The epidermis is nature's armour plate and its purpose is to keep the environment out, and keep in and protect all the important bits of the layer of skin underneath, which is known as the dermis.

The epidermis has to be a perfect combination of being impervious to the extent that it will repel the transfer of moisture, but at the same time allow the skin to breathe and sweat. It is a very carefully balanced membrane. In order for it to function perfectly, it needs an exact mix of lipids (fats), water and proteins. When this mix is at the optimum, the epidermis will be slightly acidic, and this will be indicated with a pH measurement of less than 6.

The pH of the skin also has another important effect. We have evolved over time and, as part of our evolution, we have developed a symbiotic relationship with certain bacteria, which we call flora. The flora on our skin feeds on our dead skin cells and, in return, it helps to defend our skin against certain bacteria. Among our flora is propionibacterium acnes which, when in the wrong place at the wrong time, is one of the causes of acne. This bacterium lives on, among other things, the sebaceous oils found in the follicles in the skin. In certain conditions it breeds energetically, forming the spots we call acne. If our skin is not sufficiently acidic, the acne bacteria will flourish, making us prone to acne breakouts. The first step in any acne treatment program is to ensure that the pH of the skin is acidic, allowing our flora to flourish, yet depleting the levels of acne-causing bacteria[24].

Maintaining an acidic skin is relatively straightforward. There is a hard way and an easy way. The hard way is to buy a pH meter for about £400, regularly test your skin and use low pH skin care products. Alternatively, you could do it the easy way and just use low pH products for your skin care. The easy way will also save you £400. In most cases, the pH of your skin will reflect the pH of your skin care products after about fourteen days of use. So, how does our skin become more alkaline than is desirable? The answer lies in the products that most of us use, and the biggest culprit of all is soap.

For many of us, soap is one of the defining attributes of civilisation. It enables us to separate ourselves from the barbarian by giving us control over our personal cleanliness, and allows us to choose whether or not we will be clean and fragrant. The ancient Babylonians used a soap-like material some 5,000 years ago, and its manufacture is described by the Roman chronicler

Pliny as being from tallow, a type of animal fat, and ashes. He also noted that its use was more common among men than women! However, the type of soap we commonly use today was introduced into Europe by the Moors during their occupation of Spain in the early middle ages.

Keeping clean has its challenges. Dust and dirt will wash away with water and a little effort, but the removal of grease and grime requires a little bit of chemistry. For grease to be cleaned from the skin, a substance that is both fat loving – lipophilic – and water loving –hydrophilic – must be created in order for oil and water to mix. Such a substance can be made by treating animal or vegetable fats with a strongly alkaline solution and, over the centuries, production of soap has evolved to provide us with the bars of soap and liquid gels that we know today. Regardless of price, the chemistry behind the manufacture of most soaps and gels for the face and body are fundamentally the same, and it produces an alkaline substance. If we want to maintain the acidic balance of our skin, we have to use cleansers that are specially manufactured to be acidic. Fortunately, these are becoming easier to obtain and are no longer exclusive to skin clinics. Low pH products are even available in good supermarkets, although finding them can require a good deal of patience and a powerful pair of glasses. Pears and Nutralia are examples of shower gels that are acidic, and the range is growing.

As the acidity of your skin is affected by all of the products you put on it, you can undo all the benefits of a low pH skin wash if you subsequently apply an alkaline moisturiser or sunscreen. You need to ensure that all of the products you use are slightly acidic. I would not advise putting anything on your skin that has a pH higher than six, unless there was a specific reason. Generally speaking, I would recommend using products that were between the range of pH5 to pH5.5, and these are increasingly easy to obtain from good skin clinics. Unfortunately, very few of the product ranges available from high street chemists indicate their pH balance, with the exception of some ranges promoted for oily and combination skins. If you enjoy using a product but cannot see any indication of the pH balance on the packaging, I recommend that you contact the manufacturer, most of whom will be happy to provide you with the information.

Sun protection

The next essential for good skincare is protection from ultraviolet radiation (UV). UV radiation is particularly damaging to skin. The longer wavelength UV-A, (UV type A), can penetrate into the dermal layers and, apart from increasing the risk of malignant melanomas, a dangerous type of skin cancer, it destroys newly-formed collagen. It is for this latter reason that one of the most visible signs of sun damage is a thinner skin.

Your collagen cells are living cells that will eventually die and be removed to the lymph system by macrophages, the scavenger cells in your dermis. As old collagen cells die, new collagen cells are created by another type of skin cell called a fibroblast. In the first week of their existence, the young collagen cells are exceptionally vulnerable to UV-A radiation and consequently exposure to even low levels of UV-A will cause a depletion of collagen. As the collagen depletes, the skin becomes thinner and loses its elasticity. UV-type radiation is also capable of damaging the DNA and RNA of skin cells, and this often results in more permanent types of skin damage.

The sun also causes problems with pigmentation in two very different ways. In the first instance, it can cause the permanent loss of pigmentation, a condition known as vitiligo, which has no known remedy. Alternatively, it can cause too much pigment, normally in irregular patterns, and this condition is often referred to as hyper-pigmentation.

It is important to always use a sunscreen during the daylight hours in order to avoid UV damage to the skin. More information on sunscreens is given in the next chapter; however, always use a total sunblock. Most sunscreens have an SPF rating, which is only an indication of its effectiveness in protecting against UV-B. Only a total sunblock will provide protection against UV-A. If you want a tan, you should fake it. Fake tans, both self-applied and via a spray booth, have improved enormously over the last five years and, with a little bit of experimentation, you will find one that works with your skin type to give you a convincing golden glow.

Exfoliation

The third essential element of a good skin care regime is exfoliation. Exfoliation is a process that removes dead skin cells from the surface of the skin. The immediate effect is visual; you will have a smooth and clear skin, free of most superficial irregularities.

Exfoliation will, however, substantially improve your skin if it is performed regularly. Each time you exfoliate and remove the dead skin cells, you will stimulate the skin to produce new skin cells. If this is done regularly at the correct frequency, you can restore your new skin cell production to a rate you enjoyed ten years previously, and over time your skin will thicken and superficial blemishes will begin to fade; your skin will also become more elastic and fine lines will fade away.

The critical factors to successful exfoliation are to do a little and often. To help you to do this, I have designed a peel that you can make yourself at home using everyday items that you will find in the kitchen – see *Appendix D: 'Make your own combination face peel'*. It takes five minutes to make and costs less than a cup of coffee. If you perform this treatment on a weekly basis, you will regulate your pH balance, reduce congestion and breakouts, enjoy a smooth, clear complexion and stimulate the rejuvenation process that will make your skin thicker and more elastic.

There are times, however, when good skin requires a little more help than maintaining the correct pH balance and protection from UV radiation. Your diet and exercise will feed the skin from within your body, but the skin will also benefit from topically applied treatments. We are fortunate because the cosmetic industry has made huge strides in the last decade, and creams and lotions really do what they say.

There are some simple rules to choosing good and effective products.

123

The first is that I would always recommend going to a skin clinic and having your skin professionally analysed. Often an analysis is performed free of charge with the anticipation that you will purchase any products that are subsequently recommended.

The second rule is that I would avoid spending large amounts of money on luxury brands from luxury high street stores. Luxury brands are focused on selling luxury, and the high price pays as much for marketing, packaging and presentation as it does on active ingredients.

The third rule is to avoid buying one cream that does everything, because it probably won't do any of the things particularly well. To treat the skin effectively, products should be targeted at the area of the skin they are designed to affect.

For instance, hyaluronic acid is found naturally in the dermis of the skin, and the quantity within your skin diminishes with age, resulting in reduced moisture retention and a thinner skin. A topical hyaluronic acid product needs to penetrate through the epidermis to reach the dermis, and consequently needs to have a very small molecular size to penetrate through the surface skin cells. On the other hand, a finishing moisturiser should assist the epidermis' function as a barrier to protect against the stress of the environment, and it should be designed to sit on the surface of the skin. For best effect, two separate products should be purchased and applied in layers so that the products needed to penetrate to the dermis are applied first, and the products required to stay on the surface – for instance, sunscreen – should be applied last.

Labelling

There is often confusion about the labelling of products and their ingredients. Ingredients can be described in many ways; for example, they have a name we might use in everyday conversation as well as a chemical name that describes their precise molecular structure. By example you can describe vitamin C as ascorbic acid, and vitamin E can be described as either a tocopherol or a toctrienol. Most skin care ingredients are originally obtained from very natural sources before they are then refined to give them the exact properties required; however, when you look at the list of ingredients, you will always see a list of chemical descriptions, rather than the names by which the source materials are more commonly known. The ingredients appear as a list of potentially frightening chemicals that gives no indication of their source.

All cosmetic products are required by law to list their ingredients in what is known as an INCI (International Nomenclature of Cosmetic Ingredients) list by their precise chemical description. Because we are unfamiliar with these descriptions, we are at best confused and sometimes worried about whether an ingredient is desirable or not. *Appendix C: 'Cosmetic ingredients facts, fictions and controversial ingredients'* dispels some of the more common myths and provides facts about the ingredients that cause controversy.

Some of us will want to improve our skin further and faster than can be achieved by good home care. There are also some conditions that require specialist intervention such as extensive and deep hyper-pigmentation, scars and thread veins. Over the last decade, the results of non-surgical procedures for these problems have advanced to the stage where they frequently provide a better and more enduring result than can be achieved with surgery. Non-surgical treatments are also inexpensive and normally require a little or no recovery time, so they are ideal for people with busy lives. Below is a guide to help you decide whether or not non-surgical cosmetic intervention is for you and what the treatments have to offer.

How non-surgical cosmetic treatments work

Rather than cutting, chiseling, stitching, injecting or implanting, non-surgical treatments achieve results through stimulating processes that occur naturally in your skin and body, such as:

• Stimulating collagen and elastin production to smooth and tone the skin, smoothing fine lines and wrinkles.
• Coagulating blood-based blemishes so that they naturally disappear during skin renewal.

- Stopping and controlling melanin production to tackle pigmentation blemishes.
- Massaging and stretching connective tissue to smooth atrophic scars, such as acne scars and other indentations caused by trauma.
- Metabolising deposited fat into the bloodstream, which can then be burnt off through moderate exercise.

These treatments are also reasonably painless and free from risk. They also have short recovery times.

When you choose a non-surgical clinic you should consider the following:

- Reputable non-surgical clinics will be registered with a regulatory body, which will involve an annual audit and inspection by external assessors. The Care Quality Commission (CQC) used to undertake this role, but regulations are now administered by local councils. Good clinics will have policies and protocols to ensure your safety, confidentiality and wellbeing. You can usually recognise a professional clinic by the questions you are asked. If they ask for detailed information, then it is likely that they want it in order to provide a solution specific to your needs.
- Beware of hidden costs. However, by their very nature, non-surgical treatments are unlikely to have hidden costs – i.e. no anaesthetic costs, no overnight stay or private hospital costs.
- Are the staff sympathetic? Take notice about the way that you are treated by the staff. If they don't seem interested, then they may not listen to your needs and provide you with the solution that you want.
- Do they offer free consultations? You need answers to all of your questions before you go ahead with a treatment. Some clinics charge for consultation, but even in such cases the charge is normally modest.

Facial rejuvenation and non-surgical face lifts

Non-surgical face lifts differ from their surgical alternatives by rejuvenating the skin to reverse the effects of ageing, rather than surgical and invasive intervention to manipulate the skin in its existing aged condition. Rejuvenation is not only an excellent alternative to surgery, but is also highly recommended as a first step to reversing the ageing process and delaying the need for surgery. By improving the quality of the skin, the increased tone and elasticity will restore a more youthful silhouette and will provide a resistance to wrinkles and lines. The natural radiance of rejuvenated skin, free from the ravages of age, sun and a hostile environment, will reveal a healthy vitality that cannot be achieved through surgery.

Because the treatments are focused on improving skin quality, each programme of treatments will be specific to an individual's needs and the initial condition of their skin. A treatment program would usually comprise of one or more of the following treatments:

- *Microdermabrasion* is a gentle exfoliation of the outer layer of the skin. It leaves the skin smooth, soft and radiant, and is an excellent method of rejuvenating coarse sun-damaged skin and can remove superficial scarring. Microdermabrasion stimulates the skin to naturally increase its production of collagen and elastin and, after a programme of treatments, the skin will be thicker, stronger and more elastic. The treatment is very quick and there is usually no recovery time required after the treatment. If we express the discomfort of this treatment on a toe-curling scale of one to ten, where one is almost unnoticeable and ten is a near-death experience, microdermabrasion usually rates about two.

- *Peels* achieve rapid removal of old cells in all layers of the skin using specific acids. A peel will immediately cause the skin to feel soft and smooth, and cause an immediate turnover of the skin cells. Peels are an excellent method of rejuvenating coarse sun-damaged skin and they stimulate the skin to become strong, thick and elastic. Peels frequently use a combination of salicylic, lactic and citric acids that penetrate deep into the skin, and they also are quick to perform and very safe. Normally the sensation of a peel is akin to a warm prickling feeling, and therefore they rate between three and seven on the toe-curling scale.

- *Intense Pulsed Light (IPL)* is a high-energy light therapy that reacts with pigmentation and blood in the skin. IPL treatments are sometimes referred to as photo rejuvenation. It is the treatment of choice for removing blemishes that result from sun damage. The treatment isn't exactly pain-free, but it is very quick, requiring you to grit your teeth for only a few seconds. Typical toe-curling scores for IPL treatments are between five and nine.

- *Mesotherapy* is a technique to reintroduce nutrients, amino acids, minerals and other ingredients naturally found in the skin back into skin to restore its biochemical make-up. It is a very powerful technique, and treatments can both reduce the amount of fat and restore thickness in specific areas. Mesotherapy is also capable of tightening and toning the skin and reducing wrinkles. Mesotherapy can be performed by isophoresis, which is the latest and painless technique, so you can expect a toe-curling score of about three. The scope of mesotherapy treatments is outlined in the following section.

  Body toning and sculpting treatments available using mesotherapy:

  – Targeted fat reduction is an alternative to Liposuction. Mesotherapy makes it possible to target specific areas of fat for removal. Unlike surgery, there is no mechanical removal of the fat, which has the benefit of leaving no scars, no possibility of infection and no recovery time. Mesotherapy introduces ingredients, mainly amino acids naturally found in the body, deep into the subcutaneous, or fatty, layers of the skin, which causes the unwanted fat to be metabolised. If the treatment is accompanied by a diet and a programme of exercise, the fat is burnt off and the required body shape is achieved. Good results can be achieved, and a reduction in waist measurements of six or more inches is not uncommon.

- Cellulite reduction treatments have vastly improved with the development of the new mesotherapy treatments and results can be good. Cellulite is a description of the appearance of the skin that occurs when excess fat develops under weakened layers of the skin, mainly on the thighs and buttocks of females; it also brings tears of joy to the lens of the most hardened paparazzi. Mesotherapy can tone and strengthen the outer layers of skin, while simultaneously reducing the underlying fat.
- Loose skin or skin flaps are the alternative to tummy tucks. The treatment is very successful for tightening mild to moderate loose skin, and can be used on any part of the body. The treatment involves using mesotherapy to introduce ingredients into the skin that will tighten and tone. When used for mild or moderate loose skin, the results are comparable with surgery, with the added benefit of no residual scarring.

However, prevention is always better than the cure. Good skin care will make specialist treatment less likely and, if you have had such treatments, good skin care will enhance the results and make them last longer.

The dos and don'ts of a good skin

Do:

- Keep your skin acidic. This will keep the outer layer at its most effective and keep moisture in your skin. Use Low pH cleansers and other products.
- Protect your skin from harmful ultraviolet radiation – especially UV-A – with a sunblock. It is bad, bad, bad to burn.
- Exfoliate regularly and gently. Your skin will look radiant and you will stimulate the rejuvenation process. See my recipe for a skin peel in Appendix D.
- Eat a good diet. Consume plenty of antioxidants; they protect the skin from environmental damage. Eat oily fish; they are rich in essential fatty acids. Salmon and sardines contain

DMAE, the 'wonder ingredient' that firms sagging skin. The skin responds to good nutrition. It needs good nutrition!

- Exercise. Exercise improves circulation and regulates hormones. Exercise will give you a thicker and healthier skin.
- Be happy and smile. Smiling is a great way to exercise facial muscles, and happiness keeps the dreaded hormone cortisol at bay. A study by the Max Planck Institute for Human Development in Berlin found that happy faces were judged to look younger. This makes smiling the cheapest and quickest facelift available. Try it.

Don't:

- Beware sugar! Sugar will damage skin as much as smoking and UV radiation.
- Don't smoke. If you cannot give up the weed, exhale only!
- Never use sunbeds. Sunbeds use UV-A; sunlight with all the goodness taken out. If you need a tan, use a fake tan. Modern fake tans are very good and are now available in colours other than tangerine.
- Stop frowning. It is never desirable to look miserable, and this is a facial exercise the skin doesn't need. Frowning will probably increase your cortisol levels, and that is bad news for your skin.

Essential 7:
Enjoy the sun,
nature's free tonic

By this stage, you will be highly motivated, feeling positive, mentally flexible, in optimum health and looking good. Now is the time to make life wonderful with the help of the sun.

The ancients revered the sun. It brought them light and warmth, it made the crops grow. Without the sun, there could be no life. The Egyptians worshipped Ra, the Lord of Creation and the God of the Sun and the Universe. By day, he travelled the earth in his sun boats and in the evening descended into the underworld. He created man from his tears, and pyramids were built in his honour by the Pharoahs. Today we know the sun is just a star, one of an almost infinite number of stars in the universe, although this star is rather special. The energy from our sun is our primary source of energy, without it there would be no vegetation, and without vegetation there would be no food and no oxygen. Even today it is our source of life.

We now understand that mankind was not formed from the tears of Ra, but equally we still realise that human life requires sunlight to sustain it. Apart from the essentials of food and oxygen, we know that we depend on sunlight to set our body clock, regulate hormones and strengthen our immune system.

We have also discovered that the sun equally delivers not only the means of life but also the means of death. The radiation that stimulates our production of vitamin D can at the same time cause deadly cancers (carcinomas). This awareness of the sun's sinister powers feeds our cautionary instincts and inhibits us from the pleasure of sunlight and its life sustaining benefits. In the last two decades, our increased wariness of the sun has resulted in a decrease in vitamin D levels, and this has resulted in an increase in diseases, such as rickets, that are related to a deficiency in vitamin D. It is possible, however, to have the best of two worlds. We can both enjoy the benefits of the sun and avoid the dangers.

There are very few things in life that can give us greater pleasure than feeling the warmth of the sun on a beautiful day. This is good to do; you feel wonderful and your health greatly benefits. However, the radiation of the sun not only includes the visible light that gives us daylight, but also ultraviolet radiation. It is the ultraviolet radiation that can be harmful and, as a consequence, we need to know how, why and when to protect ourselves.

Protecting yourself from ultraviolet radiation from the sun – or tanning tubes for that matter – is a little more involved than the three initials SPF (Sun Protection Factor) on tubes of sunscreen might imply. It is important we understand everything from sunblocks and sunscreens, to UV radiation and the effects of solar radiation on the human body.

The solar energy that we receive on the earth's surface is made up substantially of infrared, visible light and ultraviolet radiation. More than half of the solar energy reaching earth is the longer wavelength infrared radiation. Visible light accounts for about forty per cent of the energy, and the balance, a mere five per cent, is ultraviolet (UV).

First of all, we must learn a little about UV radiation and understand why we like to go into the sun and why it is important to go into the sun.

UV radiation - the essentials
What is UV radiation?
UV radiation is high-energy electromagnetic radiation, shorter in wavelength than visible light and just beneath blue in the visible spectrum. It is not normally visible to the naked eye, but

is absorbed by the eye, especially by the lens and the cornea. By convention, ultraviolet radiation is subdivided into three bands: UV-A, UV-B and UV-C. The shortest of the wavelengths is UV-C, fortunately for us this fatally energetic wavelength is absorbed by the atmosphere and does not reach the earth's surface. Of the two UV bands that reach the earth's surface, UV-B is the shortest wavelength and is the most energetic. UV-B will normally only penetrate into the epidermis, the outermost layer of the skin. The longer wavelength UV-A has less energy but penetrates deeper into the dermis.

Why do we need it?

UV-B radiation is needed for the production of vitamin D, which is essential for healthy bones, and a lack of this vitamin will cause rickets. Vitamin D assists the absorption of dietary calcium and phosphorus, and is also essential for a strong immune system. High levels of vitamin D are associated with lower risks for active tuberculosis, Hodgkin's lymphoma and multiple sclerosis, as well as breast, ovarian, colon, prostrate, pancreatic and other cancers.

UV radiation increases blood levels of natural opiates, feel-good chemicals called endorphins. This is why most people feel happy when in the sun.

UV-B radiation is responsible for stimulating the production of melanin, while UV-A radiation pigments the melanin. Melanin is a pigment that is used by the skin to protect the body from UV radiation. A suntan will provide a degree of protection against UV-A absorption for most people, with the exception of fair, blue-eyed people. Fair, blue-eyed people of Nordic or Celtic origins have a skin that is often referred to as Skin Type I. Their predominant melanin is a type called pheomelanin, which will not pigment to a dark brown colour, and consequently does not provide them with protection against UV radiation. This will explain why people with a Skin Type I burn rather than tan. Pheomelanin has a reddish pigment and, as UV-B stimulates further production of melanin, people with a Skin Type I go pinker rather than browner in the sun.

Sunlight regulates serotonin and melatonin production. Melatonin is a pineal hormone responsible for stimulating the circadian rhythms that control our body clock and consequently mood, energy and sleep quality. It also plays an important role in countering infections, inflammation, cancer and autoimmunity. Serotonin is a precursor of melatonin. Moderately high serotonin levels are associated with positive moods and a calm and focused outlook. Seasonal Affective Disorder (SAD) is associated with low serotonin levels.

Now let's consider the dangers of going into the sun.

Why we have to be careful

The three main forms of skin cancer – melanoma, basal cell carcinoma and squamous cell carcinoma – are largely attributed to excessive UV exposure. Skin cancer is the most common form of cancer among groups such as the white residents of Australia and New Zealand. A deadly type of skin cancer known as malignant melanoma accounts for about seventy-five per cent of deaths associated with skin cancer. According to the World Health Organisation (WHO), about 48,000 deaths from melanoma will occur each year, with Caucasian males living in sunny climates being the group most at risk. Death among males will account for about 35,000 deaths.

UV-B radiation is primarily responsible for both basal and squamous cell carcinoma which, as their name implies, are cancers that affect the epidermis. UV-B is also the radiation most associated with sunburn.

UV-A radiation is now strongly associated with melanomas, and is strongly suspected of increasing the cancer-causing effects of UV-B. UV exposure causes free radicals that damage the cell structure of the skin, and consequently visibly age the skin. Thread veins, uneven pigmentation, coarse leathery texture and actinic keratosis – scaly or crusty patches of skin – are common manifestations of sun damage.

The UV radiation that accompanies strong sunlight can damage the eyes, causing cataracts and age-related macular degeneration, and care should be taken to protect the eyes as much as the skin.

UV radiation destroys folic acid, which is essential for DNA reproduction and repair. Pregnant women with folate deficiency are more likely to give birth to low birth weight and premature infants. Folate deficiency is also associated with spina bifida, and the NHS specifically recommends that females take a daily folic acid supplement during the early stages of pregnancy.

What does this all mean?

Overall, the benefits of moderate exposure to sunshine far outweigh the risks. However, the emphasis is on moderate. To maximise vitamin D production, in Britain about two hours per week of full-body exposure to spring sunshine would suffice. That would enable a typical white-skinned person to partly – face and arms only – expose themselves for up to half an hour per day, and get all of the benefits with minimal increased risk of skin cancer. Just fifteen minutes' exposure of the retina without sunglasses is required for serotonin and melatonin regulation. For best effect, this should be as early in the day as possible. Consequently, the best advice is to expose the skin and the eyes to the sun for between fifteen to thirty minutes as early in the day as possible, certainly no longer than it takes for your skin to start going slightly pink – the first sign of burning.

Managing the risks

UV Indexing

The actual amount of safe exposure depends on the strength of the UV radiation, and this will vary enormously dependant on the location, time of year and the amount of cloud cover.

UV-A radiation is less affected by these factors and should be regarded as being dangerous between sun up and sun down at any location, regardless of the weather or time of year. Its longer wavelengths enable it to penetrate glass and, even on overcast days, eighty per cent of UV-A radiation will penetrate through the clouds.

The shorter wavelength UV-B radiation is more affected by these factors. This radiation is at its strongest between 10am and 4pm on clear days between the tropics of Cancer and Capricorn. Its strength increases with altitude and reflection from shiny surfaces such as sea, sun and snow. In Britain, it is at most potent in summer. Although UV-B accounts for less than five per cent of UV radiation, it is significantly more energetic than UV-A, and the dangers from prolonged exposure should not be underestimated.

To assist people ascertain the dangers of UV, a UV Index (also known as UVI) is published by national weather stations. The index indicates risk of damage to the skin from overexposure to the sun at specific locations, and takes into account cloud cover and other factors. The UVI is a result of predicting UV-A and UV-B radiation and making adjustments for meteorological conditions, including the ozone layer. The index is graded as follows:

UV Index	Exposure risk
0-2	Minimal
3-4	Low
5-6	Moderate
7-9	High
10+	Very High

The index is used in conjunction with skin type, classified using the Fitzpatrick Scale, to estimate how long a person can stay in the sun before there is a significant risk of sunburn.

- **Skin Type I**

Burn?	Always
Burn Time UVIndex-1:	67 minutes
Tan?	Never
Characteristics:	Celtic/Nordic
	Blue/green eyes
	Blonde/red hair

- **Skin Type II**

Burn?	Usually
Burn Time UVIndex-1:	100 minutes
Tan?	Sometimes
Characteristics:	Blonde hair
	Blue/green eyes

- **Skin Type III**

Burn?	Sometimes
Burn Time UVIndex-1:	200 minutes
Tan?	Usually
Characteristics:	White skin
	Darker hair
	Blue/brown eyes

- **Skin Type IV**

Burn?	Rarely
Burn Time UVIndex-1:	300 minutes
Tan?	Always
Characteristics:	Brown skin
	Usually brown or black hair
	Brown eyes

- **Skin Type V**

Burn?	Never
Burn Time UVIndex-1:	400 minutes
Tan?	Always
Characteristics:	Very brown skin
	Black hair
	Brown eyes

- **Skin Type VI**

Burn?	Never
Burn Time UVIndex-1:	500 minutes
Tan?	Always
Characteristics:	Afro Caribbean/Aboriginal
	Dark brown skin
	Dark brown eyes.

The UV Index is a linear scale. So a skin type III that would burn after 200 minutes when the UVI is 1, would burn after 100 minutes when the UVI is 2, and would burn after 20 minutes when the UVI is 10.

The amount of radiation indicated by the UV Index assumes that the location is at sea level and that there is a clear sky and no reflection. Burn times should consequently be adjusted to allow for the various environmental factors that will affect the UV exposure, as follows:

- 85 per cent increase from snow reflection
- 100 per cent increase above 3,000m altitude
- 25 per cent increase from white water reflection
- 50 per cent increase from still water reflection
- 20 per cent increase from sand or grass reflection
- 40 per cent increase from wet sand or wet grass reflection
- 80 per cent of UV-A passes through clouds
- 50 per cent of UV can be reflected into shaded areas

When calculating the burn time risk from UV radiation, all of the above factors should be taken into account.

For example:

a) A skin type II person sitting on a sandy beach when the UV Index is 2 will have the following burn time:
UVI 2 + 20 per cent = 2.4 = adjusted UVI.
100 minutes / 2.4 = 42 minutes burn time.

b) A skin type I person skiing in the Alps on a clear sunny day when the UV Index is 5 will have the following burn time:
UVI 5 + 85 per cent + 100 per cent = 18.5 adjusted UVI.
67 minutes / 18.5 = 4 minutes burn time.

Sun protection and Sun Protection Factors (SPF)

SPF are the initials of Sun Protection Factor and 'Factor' is the multiplier that you apply to your burn time to calculate the maximum period of time you can stay in the sun without risk of burning. So a sunscreen with an SPF of 10 when applied to the person in example A above would allow that person to be in the sun for 420 (42x10) minutes before burning, and the person in example B would be able to stay in the sun for 40 (4x10) minutes before there was a risk of burning.

To clarify the effect of using SPF sunscreens even further, if a sunscreen of SPF 50 was applied, the person in the example A would be able to stay in the sun for 2,100 (42x50) minutes – that's thirty-five hours, or all day – and the person in example B would be able to stay in the sun 200 (4x50) minutes before they had a risk of burning.

The exposure time is not increased by reapplying the sunscreen. This is important. If the skin type I person in example A above used an SPF 10 sunscreen, after fifty minutes in the sun they would not be able to reapply the sunscreen and stay another fifty minutes in the sun. The SPF gives no indication of how long the sunscreen will remain active, and it should be reapplied in accordance with supplied instructions. Generally speaking, sunscreen should be reapplied if the user has been swimming or sweating.

SPF only indicates protection against UV-B, the burning radiation. It does not indicate any protection against UV-A radiation. The concept of SPF only indicating protection against UV-B radiation harks back to the era when only UV-B was considered dangerous, because it burned skin and could be associated with carcinomas. Current thinking is that UV-A is at least as dangerous and, because there is increasing evidence to associate it with melanomas, probably more dangerous. In order to be sure of some measure of protection against UV-A, either a 'full spectrum' sunscreen – for example, Solar Moisturiser SPF30 – or a sunblock – for example, ZinClear – should be used. Unfortunately, neither the terms 'full spectrum' nor 'sunblock' indicate the level of protection provided against UV-A radiation. A star system – i.e. ★★★★★ – is gradually being introduced to indicate levels of protection, and its use will become standardised and more widespread in the next few years.

And finally...

Moderate exposure to the sun is essential for a healthy life, however over exposure can have fatal consequences. Being safe in the sun isn't all about checking the UV Index and applying the appropriate sunscreen. Lifestyle plays an important part too. The following advice won't do anybody any harm and could save their life. The more we adapt our lifestyle, the more we can enjoy and benefit from the sun.

- *Diet is important.* Fresh fruit and vegetables are essential. Go for variety, intense colours and freshness.
- *Top up folic acid.* Good foods for folic acid include broccoli, brussel sprouts, asparagus, peas, chickpeas and brown rice.
- *Antioxidants are essential.* Intensely-coloured berries and red grapes are a good source. Processed tomatoes such as tomato juice or tomato sauce will help to prevent sunburn.
- *Run to the coffee shop.* Caffeine and exercise combined will boost the body's immune system against UV radiation.
- *Dress sensibly.* Cover as much skin as possible between 10am and 4pm. Wear a hat and sunglasses.
- *Get out of the sun.* Stay in the shade when the sun is at its hottest, especially if the UV Index is 8 or above.
- *Use aftersun.* Apply antioxidant serums directly to the skin after exposure to the sun.
- *Beware UV-A.* Remember, UV-A exposure can be dangerous and is possible at any time of the day, all year in almost any location.
- *Do your research.* The UV Index is available on most major news sites on the Internet, such as www.metoffice.gov.uk
- *Don't get a tan from tanning tubes.* There are no benefits, just risks! The radiation from tanning tubes consists mainly of UV-A, the radiation associated with malignant melanomas. The amount of UV-B emitted is usually less than ten per cent of the total. Not only does UV-B cause the skin to produce vitamin D, but it also stimulates the production of the protective pigment melanin. Use fake tan if a tan is important. UV-A is the most ageing type of radiation, and a tan today will give you a tortilla skin tomorrow!

End note

The race is on to find the magic potion that will extend life, and I have no doubt that within the next ten years there will be major advances. The research into both gene therapy and stem cell therapy is showing great promise, and we are already reading press releases that give a tantalising glimpse of the future. This research is to be welcomed. However, we should be cautious; increasing the potential lifespan of a person will not necessarily improve either their life expectancy or their quality of life. Life expectancy and quality of life will continue to be very dependent on the lifestyle that we, as individuals, choose to lead.

The maximum lifespan, the greatest possible life for humans, is commonly estimated at about one-hundred-and-twenty years, a period that probably has not changed since the Stone Age. Life expectancy is different to maximum lifespan and estimates how long, according to statistics, we will probably live. For a male living in the UK it is about seventy-eight years. British women are blessed with a further five years and, on average, currently live eighty-three years. Life expectancy varies enormously, and because this variation is closely linked to lifestyle as much as access to advanced healthcare, we know that we can significantly increase our life expectancy, and quality of life, by a good lifestyle.

Once again, statistics provide valuable insight; according to the Office of National Statistics, between 2008 and 2010, men living in Chelsea – an area in London – could expect to live fourteen years longer than men living in Glasgow, Scotland's largest city. This big difference is all the more remarkable because both areas share the same healthcare system.

I like Glasgow; I have visited the city several times and enjoyed the history and the culture, and have even tried to learn the language. However, hidden away from its lovely city centre, it has severe problems, many of which are a consequence of high rates of poverty and unemployment. It has the highest murder rate in Scotland, a remarkable feat in the country with the sixth-highest murder rate in the world. Not content with having the greatest number of alcohol-related deaths, it also records the greatest number of suicides in the UK, and as if this choice of abrupt and untimely departure was not enough, Glaswegians can choose the slow road. Glasgow has been voted 'Britain's Fattest City' several years in a row.

According to a survey of 40,000 gym users by the Nuffield Health Charity, almost forty per cent of Glaswegians are obese and five per cent are morbidly obese, twenty five per cent more than any other area in the UK. The same survey revealed that thirty per cent of the inhabitants smoke and it is the fifth-worse city for sleep deprivation. 'It is a worrying problem' according to Dr. Deniszczyc of Nuffield Health, who went on to say that fat stored around the waist can contribute to significant health issues such as breast cancer and infertility. In contrast, the survey revealed that London is the fittest city.

Some other studies are specific as to the effect that certain activities, or lack of them, can have on life expectancy. Researchers from the Pennington Biomedical Research Centre in Louisiana used data collected for the National Health and Nutrition Examination Survey, which looks at health and the way of life[25]. Using data from 2005/2006 and 2009/2010, they calculated the time that people spent watching TV and sitting down. They also used data involving 167,000 adults, and concluded that life expectancy could be increased by two years if we sat for less than three hours per day, and that life expectancy could be increased by nearly one-and-a-half years by restricting TV viewing to less than two hours per day. These studies represent a few among many that show the benefits of adopting a lifestyle that improves, or at least maintains, mental and physical health and fitness.

Medical science may well soon provide us with the miracle potions and lotions that will reduce, and maybe even reverse, the rate at which our cells age. These potions, however, will not make us fit, nor will they give us the enthusiasm for life that makes awakening each morning a wonderful pleasure to be anticipated. Pills will not give us a purpose in life, nor will they bring us a positive outlook with happiness and laughter; these things, together with fulfilment and achievement, will always be the personal fruits of our individual efforts.

This book is all about improving your quality of life and life expectancy by inexpensive, easy and enjoyable adjustments to your lifestyle. It is something we are all capable of doing now, and benefiting from immediately. We do not have to wait for the pills of immortality. Health, happiness and almost eternal youth are available today.

And finally, a few more quotes from the famous:

"It takes a long time to become young."
– Pablo Picasso

"The longer I live, the more beautiful life becomes."
– Frank Lloyd Wright

"You are never too old to set another goal or to dream a new dream."
– CS Lewis

"I have enjoyed greatly the second blooming... suddenly you find – at the age of 50, say – that a whole new life has opened before you."
– Agatha Christie

Appendix A:
Glycemic Load table

The following table indicates the Glycemic Index and Glycemic Load for a range of foods that contain carbohydrates. Protein and fats have a minimal effect on blood sugar levels and consequently the glycemic load of meat, fish and most cheeses can be assumed to be insignificant. The glycemic load for leafy salads and non-starchy vegetables such as mushrooms, broccoli and spinach is negligible, and no scores are shown. The glycemic load score is the best indication of the effect a food will have on blood sugar levels.

The glycemic index shown is indicative only and is likely to vary according to such factors as variety, ripeness (for fruit and vegetables), recipe, length of cooking time etc. The glycemic index column shows the likely mean score followed by the probable range, depending on whether glucose sugar or white bread was used as the reference food, in brackets.

- Low glycemic load foods score 10 or less.
- Medium glycemic load foods score between 11 and 19.
- High glycemic load foods score 20 or more.

Food	Glycemic Index (glucose = 100)	Serving size (grams)	Glycemic Load per serving
Bakery products and breads			
Banana cake, made with sugar	47, (39-55)	80	18
Banana cake, made without sugar	55, (45-65)	80	16
Sponge cake, plain	46, (40-52)	63	17
Apple cake, made with sugar	44, (38-50)	60	13
Apple cake, made without sugar	48, (38-58)	60	9
Baguette, white, plain	57, (48-66)	30	10
Rye bread	66, (62-70)	30	6
Hamburger bun	61, (55-67)	30	9
White wheat flour bread	70, (70-70)	30	10
Whole wheat bread, average	71, (69-73)	30	9
100 per cent Whole Grain bread	51, (40-62)	30	7
Pita bread, white	68, (63-73)	30	10
Pita bread, wholemeal	56, (43-69)	50	8
Beverages			
Coca Cola®, average	58, (53-63)	250ml	15
Fanta®, orange soft drink	68, (62-74)	250ml	23
Lucozade®, original (glucose drink)	95, (85-105)	250ml	40
Apple juice, unsweetened, average	40, (39-41)	250ml	12
Cranberry juice drink	68, (65-71)	250ml	24
Grapefruit juice, unsweetened	48, (48-48)	250ml	11
Orange juice, average	50, (46-54)	250ml	15
Tomato juice, from concentrate	38, (34-42)	250ml	4

Food	Glycemic Index (glucose = 100)	Serving size (grams)	Glycemic Load per serving
Breakfast cereals and related products			
All-Bran™, high-fibre	50, (50-50)	30	12
Shredded Wheat™	83, (83-83)	30	17
Corn Flakes™, average	81, (78-84)	30	21
Weetabix™	74, (74-74)	30	16
Muesli, average	66, (57-75)	30	16
Oatmeal, average	58, (54-62)	250ml	13
Instant oatmeal (porridge), average	66, (65-67)	250ml	17
Puffed wheat, average	74, (67-81)	30	16
Cheerios™ (Kellogg's)	74, (74-74)	30	15
Special K™ (Kellogg's)	69, (64-74)	30	14
Grains			
Pearled barley, average	25, (24-26)	150	11
Sweet corn on the cob, average	53, (49-57)	150	17
Couscous, average	65, (61-69)	150	23
White rice, average	64, (57-71)	150	23
Quick cooking white basmati rice	60, (55-65)	150	23
Brown rice, average	55, (50-60)	150	18
Whole wheat kernels, average	41, (38-44)	50	14
Bulgur, average	48, (46-50)	150	12
Biscuits and crackers			
Digestives	39, (31-47)	25	6
Rich Tea	40, (35-45)	25	7
Shortbread	64, (56-72)	25	10
Rice cakes, average	78, (69-87)	25	17
Rye crackers with oats	64, (53-75)	25	10
Ryvita	69, (59-79)	25	11

Food	Glycemic Index (glucose = 100)	Serving size (grams)	Glycemic Load per serving
Dairy products and alternatives			
Ice cream, regular	61, (54-68)	50	8
Ice cream, premium	37, (34-40)	50	4
Milk, full fat	27, (23-31)	250ml	3
Milk, skim	32, (27-37)	250ml	4
Reduced-fat yogurt with fruit, average	27, (26-28)	200ml	7
Fruits			
Apple, average	38, (36-40)	120	6
Banana, ripe	49, (43-55)	120	12
Dates, dried	103, (82-124)	60	42
Grapefruit	25, (25-25)	120	3
Grapes, average	46, (43-49)	120	8
Orange, average	42, (39-45)	120	5
Peach, average	42, (28-56)	120	5
Peach, canned in light syrup	52, (52-52)	120	9
Pear, average	38, (33-42)	120	4
Pear, canned in light syrup	44, (44-44)	120	5
Prunes, pitted	29, (25-33)	60	10
Raisins	64, (53-75)	60	28
Watermelon	72, (59-85)	120	4
Beans and nuts			
Baked beans, average	48, (40-56)	150	7
Black eyed peas, average	42, (33-51)	150	13
Chickpeas, average	28, (22-34)	150	8
Chickpeas, canned in brine	42, (42-42)	150	9
Navy beans, average	38, (32-44)	150	12
Kidney beans, average	28, (24-32)	150	7

Food	Glycemic Index (glucose = 100)	Serving size (grams)	Glycemic Load per serving
Lentils, average	29, (28-30)	150	5
Soy beans, average	18, (15-21)	150	1
Cashews, salted	22, (17-27)	50	3
Peanuts, average	14, (16-22)	50	1
Pasta and noodles			
Fettucini, average	40, (32-48)	180	18
Macaroni, average	47, (45-49)	180	23
Spaghetti, white, boiled 5 min, average	38, (35-41)	180	18
Spaghetti, white, boiled 20 min, average	61, (58-64)	180	27
Spaghetti, wholemeal, boiled, average	37, (32-42)	180	16
Snack food			
M&Ms®, peanut	33, (30-36)	30	6
Microwave popcorn, plain, average	72, (55-89)	20	8
Potato crisps, average	54, (51-57)	50	11
Pretzels, oven-baked	83, (74-92)	30	16
Snickers® bar	55, (41-69)	60	19
Vegetables			
Green peas, average	48, (43-73)	80	3
Carrots, average	47, (31-63)	80	3
Parsnips	97, (78-116)	80	12
Baked potato, average	75, (56-94)	150	23
Boiled white potato, average	50, (41-59)	150	14
Instant mashed potato, average	85, (82-88)	150	17
Sweet potato, average	61, (54-68)	150	17
Yam, average	37, (29-45)	150	13

Appendix B:
Eating for energy, health and happiness

I have included a few recipes to get you started with the Immortality Diet; I hope that they can demonstrate to you that a good diet can be convenient, healthy and pleasurable, without incurring any additional cost and certainly no extra effort. There is nothing particularly special about a healthy meal, except that it should always be prepared using the best possible ingredients. This means that fruit, salads and vegetables should be fresh and ripe, and this implies they are likely to be local and seasonal. There is an added bonus to using seasonal vegetables in that it will ensure that you enjoy a variety of foods, and consequently a wide range of nutrition, throughout the year. When you buy meat, I recommend that you use a butcher who not only sources his meat locally but has also taken the trouble to find out how the animals were raised. I only buy meat that has been naturally fed, and I do this as much for taste as I do for health. Animals that graze have a depth of flavour that I have never enjoyed when eating intensively-reared meat, and my enjoyment isn't diminished by any anxieties about what else I may digesting. Good meat doesn't necessarily cost any more than the commercially-produced meat sold in supermarkets. In fact, because less popular cuts are available, you will probably be able to both eat better meat and reduce your food bill at the same time.

When I cook, I select the majority of the ingredients from the Good Food and Really Good Food categories in the diet, but I don't let strict compliance come between me a good meal.

Consequently, you will find some of the ingredients used are listed in the other categories. The important thing is to make sure that, within any given week, the majority of your food comes from the first two categories.

A handful of recipes

- The Immortals' breakfast cereal
- Pennine beef casserole
- Derbyshire roast hogget
- Easy cabbage
- Glazed carrots with garlic
- Mashed carrots and potatoes
- Red onion Yorkshire puddings
- Apple crumble (better than my wife makes)

The Immortals' breakfast cereal

This breakfast is a brilliant substitute for muesli. Because you make it yourself, you control exactly what goes into it, which is the best way of ensuring its quality. There is no sugar used, instead sweetness and complexity of flavour is obtained by using dried fruit. The dried fruit is particularly rich in antioxidants and fibre, so the flavour brings huge health benefits. The recipe also uses seeds, which add texture together with vitamins, minerals and essential fatty acids. Rolled oats provide the bulk of the mix. They are eaten raw and are slowly digested to provide a steady supply of energy throughout the day. This breakfast is a great source of fibre and protein and is packed with essential fatty acids, amino acids, antioxidants, vitamins and minerals. The complete mix, when served with full-fat milk, has a low GL score and will help to keep your blood sugar levels stable.

Ingredients:

250ml dried apricots, finely chopped
250ml dried cranberries, finely chopped
250ml dried blackcurrants, finely chopped
250ml sunflower seeds
250ml linseeds (also called flaxseeds)
250ml pumpkin seeds
Rolled oats, quantity according to taste

Method:

- Finely chop all of the dried fruit and place in a mixing bowl.
- Add the seeds to the mixing bowl.
- Mix together.
- Place in an airtight container for storage.
- Store in a cool dry place, preferably a fridge.

To serve:

Put a portion of the fruit and seed mix in a cereal bowl, add rolled oats to taste. Mix together. Add full-fat milk. Chew well.

I make a mix of the seeds and fruit and keep it in airtight containers, and only mix it with the oats when I place them both in my cereal bowl prior to eating. Some of my friends will mix in the oats when they prepare the seed and dried fruit mix. It is a matter of individual preference, and you can decide what suits you best. One of my friends grinds the linseed in a coffee grinder to ensure they are digested. You can do this too, although I don't. I believe that once the seed is ground, it rapidly oxidises and its nutritional value deteriorates. However, if you don't chew it completely, the complete seed passes straight through the gut without being digested, and this too results in no nutritional benefit. If you enjoy chewing your food, then I recommend leaving the seeds whole. For a special treat, pour some cream over the top; it is delicious and will lower the GL score even further.

Pennine beef casserole

My favourite butcher rears his own cattle, and slaughters them only when they are at their best to eat. Occasionally, when he has no meat that is fit for his butcher's block, he will shut his shop. He would rather sell no meat at all than sell something he did not know. He hangs his beef for twenty-eight days and sometimes, when he thinks he has something a bit special, he lets it hang for a little longer. His meat is the most delicious I have ever tasted. This recipe is one that I created for his shin beef. Shin beef is cut from the lower shoulder and has a gelatinous membrane woven between the fillets of meat. When cooked properly, the succulent meat melts on the tongue with a rich, satisfying flavour and the gooey sauce has the consistency of a heavenly jelly. It is food for hungry angels.

The casserole is very easy to prepare and requires little in the way of chopping or complicated mixing of ingredients. It does, however, require planning and preparation because this dish is at its best when prepared over several days. Because of this, I always make double the quantity I need so that I can put half in the freezer for later use as an emergency feast. There is quite a big list of ingredients, but these meld and mature over the cooking time to provide deep and complex flavours. You may want to add your own tweaks to make it a dish of your own. I recommend that you serve the casserole with plenty of cabbage – try my easy cabbage recipe – to make an outstandingly delicious and satisfying meal. If you want an extra touch of comfort factor, you can also serve it with my red onion Yorkshire puddings to mop up the superb gravy. This meal is completely nutritious. It contains all of the vitamins, minerals and amino acids that you need, and it is rich in antioxidants. If you use a French red wine, you will probably also digest a useful dose of resveratrol, the anti-ageing antioxidant. I should also add that the meal, even with the Yorkshire puddings, will have an extremely low GL score, so you can tuck in to your heart and stomach's content.

Ingredients:

Enough to feed six people (at least) or four rugby players (maybe).

2 kilos of shin beef, hung for at least 14 days

3 red onions

4 cloves of garlic

500g butter beans

4 medium-sized carrots

1 can of chopped tomatoes

1 bottle of red wine

1 heaped serving spoon of mixed herbs

Half a red chilli

1 serving spoon of Worcester Sauce

2 vegetable stock cubes

1 teaspoon of Marmite

Preparation – the night before:

Preparing the butter beans:

- Put 1 litre of water into a lidded saucepan, add the vegetable stock cubes and bring to the boil.
- Meanwhile, rinse the butter beans.
- When the water has boiled, stir in the stock cubes until they have dissolved, then add the butter beans to the stock.
- Bring to the boil, and then simmer gently for 20 minutes with the lid on the saucepan.
- Remove the pan from the heat and leave to stand with the lid on until the next day.

Marinating the beef:

- Cut up the beef into decent-sized chunks.
- Place into a bowl or pan.
- Add the chopped tomatoes.
- Add the wine, mixed herbs and Worcester sauce. Stir.
- Do not season with salt or pepper!
- Cover the bowl with cling film or put a lid on the pan, and leave to marinate until the next day.

Preparation – on the day:

- Allow for at least 6 hours' cooking time.
- Remove and discard the seeds from the chilli and finely chop.
- Skin the onions and chop into coarse chunks.
- Peel the garlic and finely chop.
- Put some olive oil into a large (5 litre) casserole dish.
- Add the onion, garlic and chilli and gently sauté until the onions are soft.
- Put the beef into the casserole and lightly brown the meat.
- When the meat is brown, add the wine and tomato marinade and bring to the boil.
- Once the beef is boiling, add the butter beans and any remaining stock.
- Add the marmite and return to the boil. Stir gently.
- Scrub the carrots and chop into medallions. Add the carrots.
- Do not season at this stage.
- Cover the casserole with the lid and place in an oven at 120°C (Gas Mark 1).
- After four hours, check the casserole. Stir gently, top up the liquid if necessary and return to the oven. Do not season at this stage.
- After five hours, check the casserole. Stir gently, top up the liquid if necessary and return to the oven. Adjust the seasoning with additional salt and pepper to taste.
- After six hours, remove the casserole from the oven. Make any final adjustments to the seasoning. If necessary, adjust the consistency of the sauce until it is a thick gravy; this can be done either by thinning with some beef stock (made with a stock cube) or by reducing the sauce by simmering on a hob.

To serve:

Serve with my Easy Cabbage and perhaps my Yorkshire puddings. Enjoy at leisure with favourite friends and a good bottle of red wine.Finish the meal with a good wedge of farmhouse cheddar served with Cox apples and a sweet white wine.

Derbyshire roast hogget

North Derbyshire lamb is probably one of the finest meats available anywhere in the world. The hardy sheep chew contentedly on the rugged slopes of the Dark Peak; should they look up and pause from their grazing they would enjoy one of the most splendid views in the British Isles. I am not suggesting that a good view necessarily makes good eating, but a plentiful supply of unpolluted grass and the freedom to roam makes happy, healthy sheep, and happy, healthy sheep make deliciously flavoured and wonderfully textured meat. We are particularly lucky; our neighbour rears a small flock on the hills but ten minutes' walk from our back door. In the winter, when the snow covers the surviving grass, we give her our discarded vegetables to supplement their feed. In some years, if there has been a glut of apples, there is an extra sweetness to their flavour. Our neighbour keeps her sheep over the winter, so they are known as yearlings or hogget. Hogget has a more intense and complex flavour than lamb, while retaining the succulent tenderness of the younger animal. Our hogget has less superficial fat than lamb, but it has a greater degree of marbling of fat in the flesh; this makes hogget joints very suitable for slower cooking.

When I dine out, I am always happy to be served rare, almost bloody, lamb, but I prefer to cook my hogget slower and longer to bring out the flavours. The meat will still be pink and moist, but it could not be described as rare by today's standards. I like to serve roast hogget with my easy cabbage, together with the glazed carrots with garlic. This makes a delicious meal that has all the nutrition you need; it contains all the amino acids, minerals, vitamins and antioxidants that are essential for a healthy life. It is an easy meal to prepare and cook, and while it is roasting in the oven you will have lots of opportunities to relax and share a glass of wine with friends. The meal has a very low GL score, so eat as much as you want. If there is any hogget left over, it is delicious cold. It will keep well, covered in the fridge, for about three days; however, cold hogget never survives beyond twenty-four hours in our house. This is a meat that would cause even militant vegans to salivate.

Time required: about three hours.

Ingredients:
About 2.5 kilos of leg of hogget, bone in
Mixed herbs
Wholegrain mustard
Salt and pepper.
For the gravy:
1 vegetable stock cube
1 serving spoon of Worcester Sauce
1 teaspoon of Marmite
1 serving spoon of flour
250ml red wine

Method:
* Lay out a large piece of aluminium foil, sufficient to completely wrap the joint.
* Score any thick fat on the joint to let the fat flow away when cooking.
* Cover the joint with a thin coating of the wholegrain mustard.
* Sprinkle the coated joint generously with the mixed herbs and the salt and pepper.
* Wrap the joint in the foil. The foil should meet at the top and be folded over so that it is as airtight as possible. This will keep the steam and flavours in the meat.
* Place in a roasting tin and put in the oven at 180°C (Gas Mark 4)
* Cook for 45 minutes then reduce the oven temperature to 120°C (Gas Mark 1)
* Cook for a further 60 minutes at 120°C (Gas Mark 1)
* Remove from the oven. Turn the oven back up to 180°C (Gas Mark 4)
* Remove the hogget from the foil (or vice versa). Take care not to spill any of the meat juices; you will need these for the gravy.
* Pour off all of the meat juices into a jug so that the roasting tin is dry(ish).

- Replace the joint into the tin, without the foil.
- Separate the fat from the meat juices and baste the meat with the fat.
- Return the hogget to the hot oven (180°C) and cook for a further 30 minutes.
- Remove the joint from the oven after 30 minutes. Take it out of the roasting tin and place on a carving board. Cover with foil and let the meat relax before carving.
- Now is the ideal time to start preparing the gravy.
- Pour off any meat juices from the roasting tin into the jug with juices.
- Use 100ml of the red wine to loosen any glazed meat juices stuck to the roasting dish, then pour into the jug with the juices.
- Empty the contents of the jug into a saucepan.
- Place on a hob on a low heat.
- Add the Worcester sauce, the marmite and the stock cube. Stir gently.
- Put the flour into a tumbler then add the remaining red wine (150ml).
- Mix the flour and wine into a smooth paste and add to the saucepan, stirring continuously.
- Turn up the heat of the hob and bring the gravy gently to the boil. Stir continuously.
- When the gravy boils, it will rapidly thicken. At this stage, remove from the heat and adjust the seasoning. If you require more liquid then make up some vegetable stock from a cube and add enough to reach the required consistency.
- Return to the boil just before serving.
- The meat will be ready for carving after it has stood for 30 minutes. Don't forget to drain any of the meat juices into the gravy for extra flavour.

To serve:
Enjoy this meal with a bottle of Rhone wine.
Finish the meal with my Apple Crumble.

Easy cabbage

Cabbage is a superfood that has been ruined by school cooks for generations. It is a revelation when cooked sympathetically. I use the term cabbage very broadly, and include almost any leafy green vegetable that needs to be served hot. I take advantage of the seasonal varieties that are available, and our greengrocer has a good supply of cabbage grown in the nearby counties of Lincolnshire and Cheshire. If I am travelling and pass a farm shop, I will always stop to see what is available; really fresh cabbage is a special treat.

The way to cook cabbage is to avoid using any water for anything other than washing prior to cooking. There is a lot of moisture in cabbage and this will be released as it heats. Cabbage is a very good source of vitamins, antioxidants and minerals, and many of these micronutrients are soluble in water. When you cook the cabbage in water, you will throw the nutrition away with the cooking water. Instead of water, I use a little butter to gently sauté the shredded leaves until they are soft. The aroma of cabbage cooked this way is truly stomach-seducing; unlike the unpleasant smell emitted when cabbage is boiled. Cabbage contains complex carbohydrates that release their energy as they are slowly digested. This results in a very low GL score and a minimal effect of blood sugar levels, so you can eat as much as you want. Because I am both very active and like to avoid simple and starchy carbohydrates such as potatoes, I eat big portions. Typically, I will allow half a cabbage per person. Any cabbage left over is saved for bubble and squeak, the treat of treats.

Time required: about 5 to 10 minutes.

Ingredients:

Cabbage or Spring Greens or similar

Butter (or olive oil if you prefer; salted butter will give a superior result).

Salt and pepper.

Method:

- Shred the cabbage very finely. I cut my cabbage into shreds that are almost as thin as noodles. Finely shredded cabbage requires very little cooking time and has a great texture.
- Place the shredded cabbage in fresh cold water and wash thoroughly. Change the water and repeat until the cabbage is completely clean.
- Dry the cabbage; I use a salad spinner to quickly get rid of any surplus water.
- Put a large knob of butter into a large saucepan and gently heat the pan until the butter has melted and covers the bottom of the pan.
- Place the cabbage in the pan and add another knob of butter on top of the cabbage. Grind some black pepper over the cabbage and butter.
- Cover the pan with the lid, turn up the hob slightly.
- Check the pan every minute to see if the butter on top of the cabbage has melted.
- When the butter has melted, stir the cabbage thoroughly and replace the lid.
- Every minute, check the cabbage and stir. Continue to do this until the cabbage reaches the texture you want.
- When the cabbage is wilted to your preference remove from the heat. Taste the cabbage to check for seasoning, and adjust and stir if necessary.
- Serve with a slotted spoon direct from the pan.

Glazed carrots with garlic

I find carrots very inconsistent. This is probably because I don't grow my own, and my greengrocer doesn't know a thing about them. Some days they are the sweetest most delicious things, other days they have the consistency and taste of damp fibreboard. It is hard to tell from the look of them – they all look rather orange – and it doesn't seem to make a difference whether I buy a bunch of baby carrots or a bag of battleship-sinking torpedoes. Fortunately, unless you are a rabbit, carrots require cooking if you want to release the nutrition in them; and cooking enables us to give their taste a little help. Carrots are worth eating; they are a great source of vitamins, especially vitamin A, antioxidants, fibre, minerals and complex carbohydrates. They have a low GL score, and when cooked this way they are, of course, a treat.

Time required: about 30 minutes

Ingredients:
Enough for 4 people.
4 carrots
4 cloves of garlic
1 chicken stock cube
1 serving spoon of orange juice
1 serving spoon of mixed herbs
Salted butter
Pepper

Method:
- Scrub or peel the carrots.
- Slice the carrots into strips, I quarter my carrots lengthwise. This is best done before you drink too much wine.
- Peel the garlic cloves and cut each in half.
- Place the orange juice, mixed herbs, garlic, stock cube and carrots into a saucepan.
- Add enough water to cover the carrots. Add some coarsely-ground black pepper.
- Place the pan on a hob and bring to the boil.

- Stir and reduce the heat until the carrots are simmering.
- Cover the pan with a lid and simmer for 15 minutes.
- After 15 minutes, remove the saucepan lid. Increase the heat until the carrots are gently boiling. Add a large knob of butter.
- Boil until the stock has reduced to a buttery glaze.
- Taste and adjust the seasoning according to preference.
- Serve the carrots with the glaze.

Mashed carrots and potatoes

There are times in my life when the comfort of mashed root vegetables is too appealing to be denied. In such circumstances, I always give in. Adding carrots to mashed potatoes not only adds flavour, but also increases the range of nutrition this dish provides. It is very rich in vitamins, antioxidants and carbohydrates. Adding the carrots to the mash reduces the GL score to medium and, provided that the rest of the meal has a low GL score, it will have only a moderate effect on blood sugar levels. Sometimes the wages of sin are a small price to pay for some pleasures.

I am a little eccentric when it comes to cooking potatoes. Because they are a treat, I want to enjoy them at their best, so I always cook them with their skins on and peel them afterwards. This way, the flavour and nutrition doesn't leach from the potatoes with the cooking water. I also like to prepare the mash to be ready about fifteen minutes before it is necessary; by doing this, I allow the flavours to meld and mature. I keep it in the warming oven at about 100°C (Gas Mark 1) and this restores any heat lost during the peeling and mashing process; this is important because I have grown bored with burning my fingertips when peeling the potatoes and now allow the potatoes to cool.

Cooking time: about 30 minutes

Ingredients:
Potatoes and carrots in equal measure
Butter
Salt and pepper

Method:
- Thoroughly scrub the potatoes and carrots. Do not peel or cut them up.
- Place in a saucepan and cover with water. Add salt to the water.
- Bring to the boil quickly and then reduce to a moderate boil.
- From time to time, test the potatoes and the carrots for softness. Remove any carrots and potatoes from the boiling water that

are getting soft and leave them until they are cool enough to hold.

- When the carrots and potatoes are cool enough to hold, scrape the peel off with a knife.
- Put the potatoes and carrots into a potato ricer and rice them into an ovenproof dish.
- When all the potatoes and carrots have been riced into the dish, add a large knob of butter and mash together with a fork. Add salt and pepper according to preference and continue to mash until the mixture has a creamy consistency.
- Cover the dish with foil or a butter paper.
- Place into the warm oven (100°C or Gas Mark 1) for about 10 to 15 minutes.
- Serve and enjoy.

Red onion Yorkshire puddings

There are times when I digress from the pursuit of dietary perfection. Red onion Yorkshire puddings are definitely such a digression, but the pleasure they give outweighs all guilt. I have, nonetheless, made a token attempt to reduce their GL score by using a little wholemeal flour, which gives them a little more texture. Because I make them using eggs, milk and a little onion they do have a certain nutritional value but they should be eaten solely for their sinful reward.

The ingredients are enough to fill two four-hole Yorkshire pudding trays. Any puddings left over can be successfully kept in the freezer for a couple of months.

Ingredients:

100g plain flour
50g wholemeal flour
4 eggs
200ml milk
1 red onion
Oil for cooking. I use rapeseed.
Salt and pepper

Method:

• Put the eggs, flour, salt and pepper into the bowl and beat together until you have made a smooth paste.
• Slowly add the milk while stirring the mixture.
• When all the milk has been added, beat the mixture with a whisk until you have a completely smooth batter.
• Empty the contents of the bowl into a jug.
• Chop the onions into small pieces
• Divide the onion between the Yorkshire pudding trays.
• Drizzle oil over the onion.
• Put the trays into a very hot oven, 210˚C (Gas Mark 6-7), for five minutes.
• Remove the trays from the oven.
• Pour the batter over the onion.

- Return the trays to the oven.
- Cook for 25 minutes.
- Remove the trays from the oven and serve the puddings immediately.

To serve:

These puddings have a medium GL score, so always eat them as part of a meal that includes food from the Good Food and Really Good Food categories.

They are a wonderful accompaniment for most meats, in fact anything with gravy. Enjoy them.

Apple crumble
(better than my wife makes)

Puddings are a treat reserved for the occasions when we have guests for dinner. I love having guests for dinner. I cannot offer any excuse for this blood sugar apocalypse, except that every spoonful provides a taste of heaven. The ingredients I use in the crumble mix were chosen for taste and texture; it is completely coincidental that they also help this pudding, when served with lots of double cream, to just squeeze into the moderate GL score category.

Every time I serve this desert it sparks a debate about whether a crumble is about the filling or the crumble topping. The family is evenly divided on this issue. The proportions I use seem to satisfy most, but you may wish to adjust them to suit your preferences.

The following recipe will fill a 9-inch ovenproof dish. The dish needs a lid.

Ingredients:

For the crumble topping:

75g plain flour

75g wholemeal flour

75g rolled oats

75g ground Almonds

100g unrefined cane sugar

200g butter, preferably softened.

A pinch of nutmeg

For the filling:

1 large Bramley apple

2 Cox apples

A pinch of cinnamon

Method:

First of all, make the filling:

- Wash and core the apples. I leave the peel on but you may prefer to remove it.

- Chop the apples into medium sized chunks.
- Put half of the apples and the cinnamon into a saucepan with a soup-spoon of water.
- Heat the apples until they soften into the consistency of apple sauce, then remove from the heat.
- Taste for sweetness and add more sugar if necessary.
- Put the remaining apples into the pan, mix together and set aside.

Making the crumble topping:
- Put all of the crumble ingredients into a large mixing bowl.
- Mix the ingredients together.
- Rub the mixture between the palms of your hands until the butter is completely rubbed into the mix.

Putting it together:
- Empty the apple mix into the ovenproof dish.
- Spread the crumble topping on top of the apple mixture.
- Put the lid on the dish.
- Place the dish in a hot oven (180°C or Gas Mark 4) and cook for 25 minutes.
- Take out of the oven after 25 minutes and remove the lid from the dish.
- Sprinkle some cane sugar onto the top of the crumble.
- Increase the temperature of the oven to 200°C (Gas Mark 6).
- Continue cooking for a further 15 minutes or until the top has turned golden brown.

To serve:
Serve with extra thick double cream.
Be very happy.

Appendix C:
Cosmetic ingredients facts, fictions and controversial ingredients

I have added this appendix because I encounter a lot of confusion about whether the various ingredients used in cosmetic products are harmful or beneficial. I have cross-checked the ingredients with these bodies: the American Food and Drugs Agency (FDA), the Environmental Protection Agency (EPA), and their European equivalents, the European Food Safety Agency (EFSA) and the European Medicines Agency (EMA). It not intended to be an exhaustive list of every ingredient used in every product, but rather a list of ingredients that I have been asked about in the task. All cosmetic products are required to list their ingredients by chemical description on the packaging. This, in itself, has caused a little confusion with some people who are more used to the name of the source of the ingredient. For instance, most of us can imagine what jasmine oil might be like, and it does sound rather lovely; benzyl acetate, on the other hand, certainly doesn't sound particularly lovely. They are, however, two names for the same ingredient.

Please note that most of the chemicals listed below are controversial because they can be toxic in large quantities. However, so are most things, including water. Although most are approved as being safe for cosmetic purposes, and indeed some for food purposes, they are not normally found in the skin and should be avoided unless they have a beneficial purpose. The convention for listing the ingredients in products is that they are listed in order of volume, so that any ingredient that appears first in the list will be the ingredient with the greatest volume. Generally speaking, the lower down the label that any of these ingredients occur, the lower the volume and corresponding cause for concern. An issue with some of these products is that they will appear to relieve the symptoms without tackling the cause, encouraging long-term continuous use with adverse consequences, including sensitising of the skin and allergic reaction. Solvents, including alcohol, can have a particularly adverse effect if they are used regularly on the skin. Solvents will eventually attack and break down the lipid barrier of the epidermis.

Acetone: Used as a solvent and a denaturant. It can be mildly toxic however it is naturally produced in the human body. It should only be used in a well-ventilated area and prolonged exposure should be avoided. Regarded by EPA as hazardous waste.

Alcohol: A group of organic compounds that have a vast range of forms and uses in cosmetics, especially as a thinner, solvent, astringent and preservative. In benign form, they are glycols used as humectants that help deliver ingredients into skin. When fats and oils (see fatty acid) are chemically reduced, they become a group of less-dense alcohols called fatty alcohols that can have emollient properties or can become detergent cleansing agents. When alcohols have low molecular weights, they can be drying and irritating. The alcohols to be concerned about in skin care products are ethanol, denatured alcohol, ethyl alcohol, methanol, benzyl alcohol, isopropyl alcohol, and SD alcohol, which not only can be extremely drying and irritating to skin, but also can generate free radical damage. In a product where these ingredients are at the top of the ingredient list, they will be problematic for all skin types; when they are at the bottom of an ingredient list, there is most likely not enough present to be a problem for skin.

Benzyl acetate: Can be found naturally in jasmine and other flowers. Used as a solvent and fragrance.

Benzyl alcohol: An aromatic oil found naturally in plant products. Used as a solvent, fragrance and sensitiser. Can also have an anaesthetic effect. It has safety approval for up to five per cent in personal care products and ten per cent in hair dyes.

Benzaldehyde: Used as a denaturant and fragrance. In Europe, it can be used as a flavouring in food. Can be an irritant and cause allergic reactions. It is also known as bitter almond oil and is approved for use as a flavouring agent. Exposure to skin may, in rare cases, produce allergic reactions.

Cetyl Alcohol: *See alcohol.* Cetyl alcohol (also Stearyl and Myristyl) is a fatty alcohol that keeps an emulsion from separating into its oil and water-based components. It will also stabilise foams and increase foaming capacity. Cetyl alcohol can occur naturally and is approved as a food additive.

DEA (diethanolamine): Cocamide DEA, Lauramide DEA, Linoleamide DEA, and Oleamide DEA are fatty acids found in the form of waxy solids or viscous liquids. They are used as thickening agents and foam stabilisers. They may cause the formation of carcinogenic nitrosamines when in contact with nitrosating agents and so are best avoided.

Dioxane: A solvent that is not normally added to cosmetics but can be present in small (trace) quantities as a result of the manufacturing process. Dioxane is carcinogenic at high concentrations and consequently should be avoided.

EDTA: A chelating agent that stabilises the product and inhibits unwanted changes. These products can be used as a food preserving agent.

Ethanol: *See Alcohol.*

Ethyl acetate: Also Butyl acetate. Used as a solvent. Occurs naturally (especially in apples) and is approved as a food additive.

Formaldehyde: Formaldehyde is a preservative. It is a known irritant and should be avoided where possible. Formaldehyde should not be used in aerosol products. It may cause carcinogenic nitrosamines when used in conjunction with amines – DEA, TEA, MEA.

Irritating ingredients: Some ingredients, regardless of whether they are 'natural' or synthetic, can irritate the skin and cause inflammation. In time, this inflammation can impair the immune system, break down collagen and adversely affect the skin's lipid barrier. Such ingredients are: Alcohol or SD alcohol followed by a number (Exceptions: ingredients such as cetyl alcohol or stearyl alcohol are standard, benign, wax-like cosmetic thickening agents and are completely non-irritating and safe to use; SD alcohols are not considered a problem when they are used in minute amounts, as is the case with some ingredient mixtures.), Ammonia, Arnica, Balm mint, Balsam, Bentonite, Benzalkonium chloride (if it is one of the main ingredients), Benzyl Alcohol (if it is one of the main ingredients), Bergamot, Camphor, Cinnamon, Citrus juices and oils, Clove, Clover blossom, Coriander, Cornstarch, Essential Oils, Eucalyptus, Eugenol, Fennel, Fennel oil, Fir needle, Fragrance (may be listed as "Parfum"), Geranium, Grapefruit, Horsetail, Lavender, Lemon, Lemongrass, Lime, Linalool, Marjoram, Melissa (lemon balm), Menthol, Menthyl Acetate, and Menthyl PCA, Mint, Oak bark, Orange, Papaya, Peppermint, Phenol, Sandalwood oil, Sodium C14-16 olefin sulphate, Sodium lauryl sulphate, TEA-lauryl sulphate, Thyme, Wintergreen, Witch hazel, Ylang-ylang.

Isopropanol: *See alcohol.* Isopropanol is a derivative of petroleum used in antifreeze. It can be used as a solvent for essential oils. It is best avoided.

Lanolin: Lanolin is an oil or wax derived from sheeps wool and is widely used in cosmetics and the food industry (chewing gum). Lanolin is a well-tested moisturiser suitable for dry skins. There is a very small risk of sensitisation.

Limonene: A natural fragrance ingredient. It is associated with contact dermatitis, and some research associates it with the growth of tumours. It is best avoided.

Linalool: Linalool is a naturally occurring substance (from lavender and coriander) used for fragrance and flavours. Its use is restricted because of potential sensitisation. When exposed to air, it can be an irritant and an allergen and is best avoided.

Menthol: Menthol is derived from peppermint. It has anti-microbial and anaesthetic properties and is also used for its fragrance. It can be an irritant and have a sensitising effect.

Natural Ingredients: All of the following natural ingredients can cause skin irritation, allergic reactions, skin sensitivity, and/or sun sensitivity: Almond extract, Allspice, Angelica, Arnica, Balm mint oil, Balsam, Basil, Bergamot, Cinnamon, Citrus, Clove, Clover Blossom, Cornstarch, Coriander oil, Cottonseed Oil, Fennel, Fir Needle, Geranium Oil, Grapefruit, Horsetail, Lavender Oil, Lemon, Lemon balm, Lemongrass, Lime, Marjoram, Oak bark, Papaya, Peppermint, Rose, Sage, Thyme, Witch Hazel, Wintergreen.

Parabens: Parabens are a group of preservatives that are used for their preservative properties, they prevent the growth of bacteria and fungi. They can have a weak estrogenic effect, which may be a cause for concern; however parabens are 100,000 times weaker than natural estrogens in the body.

PEG: PEG is polyethylene glycol that is used as a used as a stabiliser and delivery agent.

Petrolatum: Petrolatum is a pale yellow or colourless semi-solid derived from mineral oil and is more frequently referred to by the brand name Vaseline. Petrolatum is used to provide a protective barrier on the skin. It is very stable and inert and has very little effect on the skin other than providing a barrier that protects it from the environment and enable it to retain moisture.

Phthalate: Phthalates are used as solubulisers, plasticisers and denaturants. Phthalates are very controversial and certain types are banned in some countries. There are three types of phthalates that may be found in cosmetics: Diethyl Phthalate (DEP), Dimethyl Phthalate (DMP) and Dibutyl Phthalate (DBT). DBT is banned in Europe and has been shown to be a reproductive and developmental toxin. There is suspicion that exposure in early pregnancy may cause problems to the reproductive system of a foetus (especially boys) and subsequently should be avoided while research continues.

PPG: Polypropolene Glycol (PPG) attracts water and is used as a humectant for moisturisers. PPG is also used to stabilise products against extreme heat and cold. It is also used as a delivery medium. PPG is also permitted as an indirect food additive.

Propyl: See Alcohol. Propyl (also isopropyl) alcohol is found in many over-the-counter products and inhibits microbial growths and extends shelf life. It has a cooling effect on the skin when evaporating and has an antiseptic effect. It is used as a thinner and stops products foaming. It is also used as a food additive.

Soy: Soy extract is used as an antioxidant and an anti-inflammatory agent. Genistein is a component of soy and has a stimulating effect on collagen. Although when consumed as a food, soy may have an estrogenic effect there is no evidence this applies when applied topically.

Sulphur: Sulphur is an antibacterial agent. However it also has a high pH which can encourage the growth of certain bacteria on the skin.

Talc: Talc is also known as French Chalk and is a naturally occurring silicate mineral. It is used to absorb moisture and oil.

TEA: Triethanolamine (TEA) is used as a pH balancer. It is only approved for discontinuous use and should always be rinsed off the skin. It may cause carcinogenic nitrosamines when used in conjunction with amines – DEA, TEA, MEA.

Urea: Urea (sometimes known as carbamide) is used in cosmetics for its water binding and exfoliation properties, and also as a pH stabiliser. It can be irritating to the skin in large quantities.

Appendix D:
Make your own combination face peel

This peel is an ideal way to gently exfoliate the skin. Exfoliation is a process that removes the dead skin cells that form the outer layer of the skin, known as the stratum corneum. This treatment will decongest the surface of the skin and stimulate the production of new skin cells. The result will be a smoother, clearer, more vibrant complexion and a thicker, more youthful-looking skin.

The combination peel uses a variety of acids that are easily available from natural sources. The use of different acids enables the peel to penetrate to different depths of the skin; this increases the exfoliating effect and enhances the stimulation of skin cell production. The combination of these attributes makes this peel ideal for controlling breakouts, treating minor sun damage and slowing the effects of ageing. This peel is safe for all skin types, but do not use it if you are sunburnt or you intend to go into strong sunlight within 48 hours.

This peel will be less aggressive than a peel you might have at a skin clinic, however it will be as strong as a typical peel you might receive at a beauty salon. It is important that you exercise caution when using this peel, and it is your responsibility to satisfy yourself that you both understand and are happy with the reaction you experience.

When using this peel for the first time, you will need to test for allergic reaction and sensitivity; neither of these reactions is likely as the products used are commonly consumed without incident. The full formulation does, however, contain salicylic acid and if you are allergic to any type of salicylic or aspirin you should omit the aspirin from the recipe. You can test for an allergic reaction by using a cotton bud to dab a very small amount of the peel mixture on one ear lobe and waiting for ten minutes. If you suffer from eczema, asthma or have any other allergies, you should extend the waiting time to thirty minutes. After the allotted time, or the instant any adverse reaction occurs, the peel should be washed off with plenty of tepid water. It is very unlikely you will have any adverse reaction (i.e. swelling, increased pulse or discomfort) but if you do, these symptoms should rapidly disappear within a few minutes; if they persist, you should visit your doctor. You can test for sensitivity by applying the peel for a short period of time. This is explained in the instructions for use.

Glycolic, citric, lactic and salicylic acid peel

To make the peel, you will need:

A small bowl

The freshest lemon you can find. Light yellow lemons are preferable to dark yellow as they are more acidic

Six uncoated aspirin tablets

Two heaped soup spoons of pure cane sugar

A large spoonful (20ml) of Greek yoghurt

Method:

• Take the aspirins and grind them into fine powder. You can use a pestle and mortar or use two teaspoons to do this. The ground aspirin should be placed into the bowl.

• Extract 20ml of juice from the lemon and place into the bowl.

• Add the sugar into the bowl.

• Mix the aspirin, the sugar and the juice together until it forms a solution.

• Add the yoghurt.

• Mix the ingredients thoroughly until most of the sugar is dissolved. It is acceptable if the mixture feels a little gritty.

• Now make some neutraliser:

• The purpose of the neutraliser is to neutralise the reaction if it feels out of control, and it should only be used for this purpose. Once you have experienced the peel and have confidence in the reaction, you can dispense with this precaution.

• Make the neutraliser by adding a heaped teaspoon of baking soda to 100ml of water in a glass and stir into a solution.

Applying the peel:

• Using the tips of the fingers, apply the peel solution to the face with a gentle circular action. Avoid the eyes. If the peel comes in contact with the eyes, you must immediately apply some neutraliser with a cotton bud until all the acid has been removed from the area. Do not use too much pressure when applying the peel. You may also apply the peel to the neck and the back of the hands and any other area you may want.

- If this is your first peel, you should terminate it after one minute. The peel is terminated by thoroughly rinsing the treated area with tepid water.
- If you feel extreme discomfort, the peel should be terminated using the neutraliser. After the reaction has disappeared, the area should be rinsed with plenty of tepid water.
- If there is no lasting sensitivity or irritation from your first peel, your second peel should be terminated after 5 minutes.
- You should not have any further peels if you experience any sensitivity or irritation from the second peel that lasts for more than 48 hours.
- After your second successful peel, you can apply any peel solution remaining in the bowl once the first application feels dry to the touch.
- Your third peel should be terminated after 10 minutes.
- The duration of subsequent peels can be extended to 15 minutes.
- The ideal frequency for the peels is one peel per week. I do not recommend that you treat yourself more frequently. You should extend the interval between treatments if you find your skin is taking longer to recover from the peel.
- Dry the skin thoroughly after the peel is terminated. Apply moisturiser and sun block.

Please note that your skin will be more susceptible to sunburn for at least 48 hours following the peel. During this period, you should avoid direct sunlight and always wear sun block during daylight hours – even indoors.

Appendix E: Glossary

The following definitions are relevant to the context in which these words are used in this book. Other definitions, for other contexts, will undoubtedly exist elsewhere.

By and large, the glossary contains definitions for words and expressions that are not listed in the contents section at the beginning of the book.

Aerobic: A type of low or moderate intensity exercise that relies of the use of oxygen for the release of energy into the muscle. Aerobic exercises are usually performed over an extended period of time, and are sometimes referred to as cardio exercises.

Alzheimer's Disease: Alzheimer's is the most common form of dementia and its symptoms include problems with memory, reasoning and behaviour. Alzheimer's is a progressive disease.

Antioxidants: as used by nutritionists are molecules that neutralise 'free radicals'. They prevent these free radicals from rampant oxidation, which may damage other molecules, particularly DNA and other nucleic acids.

Cardiovascular: An expression for the heart and the blood vessel system of arteries and veins. Cardiovascular diseases are the biggest cause of adult death worldwide.

Circadian Rhythm: A cycle of the physiological processes of living things. This cycle is normally approximately twenty-four hours long and can be influenced by external factors such as temperature and sunlight.

Conscious: For the purposes of this book, this term refers to that part of our mind or thoughts that we are aware of, and that we directly control. *See subconscious.*

Cortisol: A hormone that is released in response to stress. It is often called the 'flight or fight' hormone. Its purpose is to increase blood sugar and aid fat, protein and carbohydrate metabolism. Cortisol also suppresses the immune system and long-term overproduction will result in reduced bone formation. It is essential to the body; however, elevated levels are detrimental in the long term.

Dementia: A general term for a decline in mental capability that is sufficiently severe to affect daily life. Alzheimer's disease accounts for around seventy per cent of all cases of dementia; vascular dementia, which occurs after a stroke, is the second most common type of dementia.

Endocrine hormone: A hormone that is secreted directly into the bloodstream by glands.

EPA (Eicosapentaenoic Acid): A polyunsaturated fatty acid that is found in fish oil or oily fish such as salmon, mackerel and sardines. These oils can be referred to as Essential Fatty Acids (EFA); however not all EFAs are EPAs.

Epidemiology: The study of health in defined populations. Epidemiology looks for associations between health-influencing events and their possible effects on health within the population.

Epidemiologist: Someone who undertakes epidemiological studies. A famous epidemiologist was Dr. John Snow, who investigated cholera epidemics in the nineteenth century. He noticed that cholera outbreaks were clustered around certain water pumps, especially one in Broad Street, Soho. To test his assumption that cholera was caused by water from the well, he added chlorine to the water and removed the handle to the pump.

The outbreak of cholera ended and the science of epidemiology was born.

Essential Fatty Acids: Essential Fatty Acids are fatty acids that the body obtains from diet because it is unable to synthesise them. These fatty acids can be used for biological purposes as well as the supply of fuel. Fatty acids can be either saturated or unsaturated, terms that refer to their chemical composition, and they are produced when fats break down.

European Union: A confederation of twenty-seven states, most of which are in Europe. Britain's entry was probably due to the difficulty, during the 1960s at least, of finding a decent restaurant west of Calais, and the very strict regulations that then existed restricting the amount of money that could be taken east of Dover.

Glycation: a process where sugar reacts with proteins such as collagen in the skin, which restricts the nutrition available to the skin cells.

Goals: Goals are the things you wish to achieve and are the focus of your motivation. Goals can be the overall goals that you wish to achieve in your life, sometimes referred to as prime life goals, and are the manifestation of what health, happiness and abundance mean to you. Goals can also be more immediate, for example, the things that you wish to achieve today or this week.

HMRC: An abbreviation for Her Majesty's Revenue and Customs. Benjamin Franklin reputedly said that nothing is so certain in life as death and taxes. I should add that the two types of people that will always be involved with your life, other than your parents, are undertakers and taxmen.

Incentive: An external reward for undertaking a task that is not intrinsically related to the task.

Life expectancy: The expected, or probable, period of life. This varies according to healthcare and lifestyle. The lowest life expectancy occurs, unfortunately, in Africa and reflects very high rates of infant mortality. The highest life expectancy occurs in Japan.

Lifespan: Total period of life, from birth to death. The maximum lifespan of humans is about 120 years. Jeanne Calment, a French woman, lived for 122 years and 164 days.

Marmite: A dark, sticky substance that has a taste that is very hard to describe other than it is salty and malty. It is excellent on buttered fingers of bread, which are known as soldiers. In Australia you can buy a similar food called Vegemite

Motivation: The inner force or drive that enables a person to choose and undertake various activities, and provides the reward of satisfaction when those tasks are being undertaken.

Negative: An outlook or frame of mind that stops you from anticipating good outcomes from your, and probably everyone else's, actions. A negative outcome restricts your belief that you can positively influence your life. Some negative people are often referred to as energy vampires; these people stalk people with a positive outlook in order to suck the life force out of them. However, you can repel them by winking at them.

NLP: Neuro Linguistic Programming is a process or technique of using both the subconscious and conscious parts of the mind to achieve positive outcomes.

Palaeolithic: A term used to describe the time when ancient stone implements were used, or the 'Stone Age' in common parlance. A Palaeolithic diet is consequently the diet enjoyed by our Stone Age ancestors and consisted of things that could be either picked or caught and then eaten without fatal consequences.

Plastic Surgeons: Surgeons who have received specific training in Aesthetic Surgery. Plastic Surgeons are on the Specialist Register of Plastic Surgeons maintained by the General Medical Council. You can check whether a surgeon is on the Specialist Register by telephoning the General Medical Council Registry line on 0161 923 6602.

Polyunsaturated Fatty Acids: Fatty Acids that include omega-3, omega-6 and omega-9. I will avoid the chemistry, but polyunsaturated acids supply energy to muscles and organs and also aid in the formation of cell membranes.

Positive: An outlook or frame of mind that enables you to anticipate the good outcome and benefits of your actions and enjoy happiness.

Posture: A frame of mind that affects thoughts, behaviour and physical bearing. Adopting a posture can be assisted by changing your physical bearing to reflect the required frame of mind.

Subconscious: The mind other than that part of the mind that is actively engaged in current, or conscious, reasoning, calculation or thinking. It is that part of the mind where activity, that we are not aware of, is taking place outside of our direct control and in the background, such as controlling breathing, walking, heartbeat and balance. This can be alternatively called the unconscious mind; however, I have avoided this term to avoid confusion with the consequences of drinking too much wine.

Reticular Activating System (RAS): A part of the brain that monitors all of the information that the brain is processing, and alerts the conscious mind when the information is relevant for immediate action or consideration; for example, when danger is detected.

Trigger: A sight, sound, touch, memory event or other thing that can precipitate a positive, confident and happy emotion.

Try: A very bad word. Never use it.

Values: Values are the ethical principles by which you judge the actions of yourself and others, such as honesty and loyalty.

Vitamins: Nutrients that we require from our diet in very small amounts that are essential for the functioning and maintenance of cells and other biological functions.

Appendix F: References

I have kept references to a minimum. This book is intended to stimulate thought rather than act as a reference book, and the flow of reading can be disturbed by constant referral to the source details. I have taken great care in researching all of the information presented to you, and have only provided references where the supporting research may be hard to find using internet search engines. The information on nutrition has been checked against at least two reputable sources, for instance the NHS, European and American Public Health organisations.

Essential 2: The power of being positive

1   Steptoe,Wardle, Marmot. 'Positive affect and health-related neuroendocrine, cardiovascular, and inflammatory processes', Whitehall II study, Proceedings of the National Academy of Sciences 2005.

2   Steptoe, Wardle. 'English Longitudinal Study of Ageing', Proceedings of the National Academy of Sciences, 2011.

3   Shawn Talbot 'The Cortisol Connection', Hunter House. June 2007.

4   Julian Martins, Journal of the American College of Nutrition, October 2009. vol 28, No 5 525-542.

5   'Eliminating diabetes and depression, and boosting education, most likely to ward off dementia.' British Medical Journal, August 2010

6   Jacka, 'Red Meat Consumption and Mood and Anxiety Disorders'. Journal of Psychotherapy and Psychosomatics. 2012.

7   D Carney, Cuddy, and Yap. 'Power Posing: Brief Nonverbal Displays Affect Neuroendocrine Levels and Risk Tolerance', Psychological Science , 2010

Essential 3: Flexing the mind
8   'Eliminating diabetes and depression, and boosting education, most likely to ward off dementia.' British Medical Journal, August 2010
9   Val Gilbert. 'The Daily Telegraph - 80 Years of Cryptic Crosswords'. November 2004
10   Williamson, Feyer; 'Moderate sleep deprivation produces impairments in cognitive and motor performance equivalent to legally prescribed levels of alcoholic intoxication', British Medical Journal, October 2000
11   Harrison & Horne. 'The Impact of Sleep Deprivation on Decision Making: A Review', Journal of Experimental Psychology, Vol 6, No 3,236-249. 2000
12   Basheer, Strecker, Thakkar. 'Adenosine and sleep-wake regulation'. Harvard Medical School, 2004 Aug;73(6): 379-96.
13   Kripke, Garfinkel, Wingard, Klauber, Marler. (2002) Archives of General Psychiatry, vol 59, p131
14   Duffy, Cain, Chang. 'Sex difference in the near-24-hour intrinsic period of the human circadian timing system', Proceedings of the National Academy of Sciences, 2011-09-13 vol 108, p15602
15   'The rhythms of life', New Scientist Magazine, Oct 2011, p42

Essential 4: Importance of the Body
16   Metcalfe, Babraj, Fawkner, Vollaard, 2012. 'Towards the minimal amount of exercise for improving metabolic health: beneficial effects of reduced-exertion high-intensity interval training', European Journal of Applied Physiology, 112(7), pp. 2767-2775. DOI: 10.1007/s00421-011-2254-z

Essential 5: Eating for Health

17   National Library of Science (US); Profiles in Science, Linus Pauling

18   Ledesma,Munari et al. 'Monounsaturated fatty acid (avocado) rich diet for mild hypercholesterolemia', Archives of Medical Research (1996 Winter) 27(4):519-23

19   Chavarro, Rich-Edwards, Rosner,Willet 'A prospective study of diary food intake and anovulatory infertility', 2007. Human Reproduction 22(5); 1340-7

20   Mozaffarian et al. 'Trans-Palmitoleic Acid, Metabolic Risk Factors, and New-Onset Diabetes in U.S. Adults', Annals of Internal Medicine, December 21 2010.

21   Lansley, Winyard et al, 'Acute Dietary Nitrate Supplementation Improves Cycling Time Trial'; Medicine and Science in Sports & Exercise, June 2011, 43-6

22   Dr Jiali Han et al. 'Coffee Consumption Inversely Associated With Risk of Most Common Form of Skin Cancer', Cancer Research. July 1, 2012.

Essential 6: Looking the part

23   Plastic Surgeons are surgeons who have received specific training in Aesthetic Surgery. Plastic Surgeons are on the Specialist Register of Plastic Surgeons maintained by the General Medical Council. You can check whether a surgeon is on the Specialist Register by telephoning the General Medical Council Registry line 0161 923 6602.

24   Schmid, Korting 'The concept of the acid mantle of the skin: Its relevance for the choice of skin cleansers', Dermatology 1995 191:276-280

End Note

25   Katzmarzyk, Min-Lee. 'Sedentary behaviour and life expectancy in the USA: a cause-deleted life table analysis', BMJ Open2012;2:e000828 doi:10.1136/bmjopen-2012-000828

2676493R00107

Printed in Great Britain
by Amazon.co.uk, Ltd.,
Marston Gate.